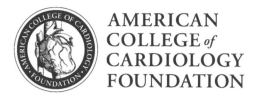

AMERICAN
COLLEGE *of*
CARDIOLOGY
FOUNDATION

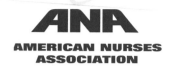

AMERICAN NURSES
ASSOCIATION

CARDIOVASCULAR NURSING:
SCOPE AND STANDARDS
OF PRACTICE

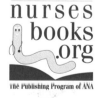

nurses
books
.org

The Publishing Program of ANA

AMERICAN NURSES ASSOCIATION
SILVER SPRING, MARYLAND
2008

Library of Congress Cataloging-in-Publication data

Cardiovascular nursing: scope and standards of practice.
   p. ; cm.
   Includes bibliographical references and index.
   ISBN-13: 978-1-55810-259-0 (pbk.)
   ISBN-10: 1-55810-259-0 (pbk.)

RC
674
.C366
2008

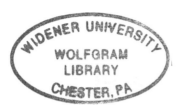
The American Nurses Association (ANA) is a national professional association. This ANA publication— *Cardiovascular Nursing: Scope and Standards of Practice*—reflects the thinking of the nursing profession on various issues and should be reviewed in conjunction with state board of nursing policies and practices. State law, rules, and regulations govern the practice of nursing, while *Cardiovascular Nursing: Scope and Standards of Practice* guides nurses in the application of their professional skills and responsibilities.

Published by Nursesbooks.org
The Publishing Program of ANA

American Nurses Association
8515 Georgia Avenue, Suite 400
Silver Spring, MD 20910-3492
1-800-274-4ANA
http://www.Nursesbooks.org/

ANA is the only full-service professional organization representing the nation's 2.9 million Registered Nurses through its 54 constituent member associations. ANA advances the nursing profession by fostering high standards of nursing practice, promoting the economic and general welfare of nurses in the workplace, projecting a positive and realistic view of nursing, and lobbying the Congress and regulatory agencies on healthcare issues affecting nurses and the public.

Design: Scott Bell, Arlington, VA ~ Freedom by Design, Alexandria, VA ~ Stacy Maguire, Sterling, VA ~ *Composition*: House of Equations, Inc., Arden, NC ~ *Editing*: Steven A. Jent, Denton, TX ~ *Proofreading*: Ashley Mason, Atlanta, GA ~ *Printing*: McArdle Printing, Upper Marlboro, MD

First printing April 2008.

ISBN-13: 978-1-55810-259-0   SAN: 851-3481   3M   04/08

ACKNOWLEDGMENTS

This document was developed by a Task Force of Cardiovascular Nursing Organization Representatives whose collaborative efforts were vital to the development of a scope and standards for cardiovascular nursing that represents the diversity of practice today. The members of the task force gratefully acknowledge the support of the American College of Cardiology Foundation in facilitating the collaboration for this document. The Scope and Standards Task Force would like to give thanks to Carol J. Bickford, PhD, RN-BC, Senior Policy Fellow, Department of Nursing Practice and Economics, for her guidance in the development of the *Cardiovascular Nursing: Scope and Standards of Practice.*

Scope and Standards Task Force Members
- Eileen Handberg, PhD, ARNP-BC, FAHA (Chair)
- Nancy M. Albert PhD, CCNS, CCRN, CNA, FAHA
- Angela P. Clark, PhD, RN, CNS, FAAN, FAHA
- Paula Feeley-Coe, MSN, RN, CCTC
- Jonni Cooper, PhD, MBA, BSN, CVRN
- Kenneth A. Gorski, RN, RCIS, FSICP
- Meg Gulanick, PhD, APRN, FAAN, FAHA
- Melanie T. Gura, MSN, RN, CNS, FHRS, FAHA
- Patricia A. Matula, MSN, RN
- Robin E. Rembsburg, PhD, APRN-BC, FNGNA, FAAN
- Barbara Riegel, DNSc, RN, CS, FAAN
- Mary Rummell, MN, RN, CPNP, CNS
- Kristen Sethares, PhD, RN
- Julie Stanik-Hutt, PhD, ACNP, CCNS
- Robin J. Trupp, PhD(c), MSN, ACNP-BC, CCRN, CCRC, FAHA
- Kathleen K. Zarling, MS, APRN-BC, FAACVPR

Scope and Standards Reviewers

Douglas Beinborn, MA, BSN
Barbara J. Fletcher, MN, RN, FAHA, FAAN
Erika S. Froelicher, PhD, RN, FAAN, FAHA
Suzanne Hughes, MSN, RN, FAHA
Jane A. Linderbaum, MS, FNP
Kathleen McCauley, PhD, RN-BC, FAAN, FAHA
Ellen Strauss McErlean, MSN, RN, FAHA, CNS
Elizabeth Tong, MS, RN, CPNP, FAHA, FAAN

American College of Cardiology Foundation Staff Liaisons

Christina A. Chadwick, MSN, RN
Brenda Dorick-Miller, MSN, RN
Marcia Jackson, PhD

American Nurses Association (ANA) Staff

Carol J. Bickford, PhD, RN-BC—Content Editor
Yvonne Humes, MESA—Project Coordinator
Theresa Myers, JD—Legal Counsel

Endorsing Organizations

Descriptions and websites of these groups are in Appendix A, which begins on pg. 45.

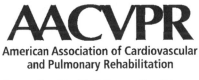

American Association of Cardiovascular
and Pulmonary Rehabilitation

Promoting Health & Preventing Disease

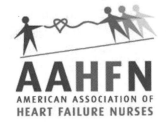

AMERICAN ASSOCIATION OF
HEART FAILURE NURSES

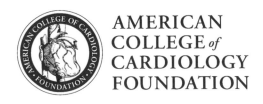

AMERICAN
COLLEGE *of*
CARDIOLOGY
FOUNDATION

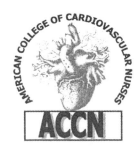

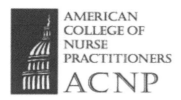

AMERICAN
COLLEGE OF
NURSE
PRACTITIONERS
ACNP

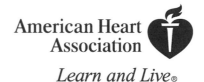

American Heart
Association

Learn and Live®

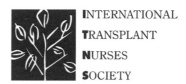

Heart Rhythm Society
Restoring the Rhythm of Life

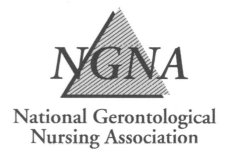

INTERNATIONAL
TRANSPLANT
NURSES
SOCIETY

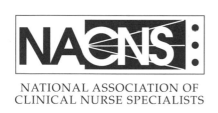

NATIONAL ASSOCIATION OF
CLINICAL NURSE SPECIALISTS

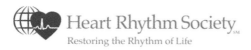

National Gerontological
Nursing Association

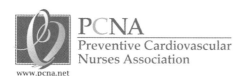

PCNA
Preventive Cardiovascular
Nurses Association
www.pcna.net

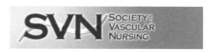

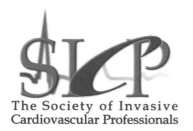

The Society of Invasive
Cardiovascular Professionals

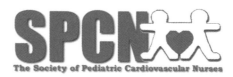

CONTENTS

INTRODUCTION

Cardiovascular disease is the primary cause of death and disability in men and women worldwide. Cardiovascular disease is responsible for over 36% of all deaths in America. Nearly 80 million adults in the United States are currently living with some form of cardiovascular disease. An estimated 37 million of these are 65 years or older. One out of every 85 babies is born with a congenital heart defect, which is now the major cause of birth-defect-related deaths. The number of people with severe congenital heart disease has risen by 85% in adults and by 22% in children over the past 15 years. Diseases of the cardiovascular system are responsible for much of the economic burden of health care in the United States and other developed countries. The estimated medical and disability cost for treatment of cardiovascular diseases in 2007 is $431 billion (AHA 2007).

Over the past 60 years, nurses have been key members of teams providing care for patients with cardiovascular health needs in a wide variety of healthcare environments. Heart surgery began in 1944 with the first palliative procedure for "blue" babies. The first open heart surgery was performed in 1955 to repair a congenital defect. In the 1950s nurses helped develop specialized operating rooms for heart and lung surgery and cardiac catheterization laboratories. In 1957, one of the world's first coronary care units (CCUs) opened in America. At that time the units were called "heart rooms" or constant care units because nurses provided care around the clock for these vulnerable patients. Both surgical and post-myocardial infarction patients were treated in this environment. Coronary care units provided a model for specialized care where nurses learned about arrhythmia recognition and early defibrillation. Infants and children were typically isolated in specialized areas of pediatric wards, whose nursing staff acquired high levels of skill in yet another important area of cardiovascular health care. As the science of cardiovascular nursing emerged, expectations of care rose among the public, patients, and the healthcare professions.

Today, the field of cardiovascular nursing is exciting and rich with opportunities for nurses to affect the lives of countless patients and families. Nursing practice encompasses the vast needs of patients across the lifespan, from newborns and children to the elderly. Given the prevalence of people who are living with preventable cardio-vascular conditions that are now chronic and debilitating, cardiovascular nurses are in a unique position to create prevention programs for individuals and communities. Preventing cardiovascular disease starts in infancy. Helping people avoid obesity, stop smoking, be more active, and eat healthier can significantly reduce morbidity and mortality associated with cardiovascular disease. Cardiovascular nurses can and do lead many of these prevention efforts.

Excellence in cardiovascular nursing requires advanced cardiovascular knowledge and skills. This document describes this knowledge base, and thereby provides a framework for developing educational curricula and establishes standards of practice for cardiovascular nurses.

CARDIOVASCULAR NURSING SCOPE OF PRACTICE

Definition of Cardiovascular Nursing

Cardiovascular (CV) nursing is specialized nursing care focused on the optimization of cardiovascular health across the lifespan. This care includes prevention, detection, and treatment of cardiovascular disease in individuals, families, communities, and populations of all ages. Cardiovascular health is reflected in a lifestyle or environment that prevents or delays the development or progression of cardiovascular disease.

Cardiovascular nurses are registered nurses who emphasize health promotion, disease and injury prevention, symptom recognition, disease management, and self-care knowledge and adherence in order to improve patient outcomes. Cardiovascular nursing uses evidence-based practice to improve patient functional capacity and quality of life, and to enhance the heart health of communities. Cardiovascular nurses develop, implement, and participate in nursing and multidisciplinary cardiovascular research to advance the prevention, diagnosis, and treatment of cardiovascular disease. Practice-based research by cardiovascular nurses provides a better understanding of the impact of healthcare practices and nursing interventions on patient outcomes.

Key elements of cardiovascular nursing care include the development of programs that promote heart health: the education and counseling of individuals, families, and communities about heart health; interventions, such as exercise, that maintain or improve physiologic, psychological, and psychosocial homeostasis; interventions that facilitate and optimize behavioral change and treatment adherence over time; and advocacy to support patients and families during the planning, implementation, and evaluation of their care.

Cardiovascular nurses also focus on optimizing the manner in which health care is delivered in order to provide exceptional cardiovascular care. Cardiovascular care at the healthcare delivery level emphasizes quality monitoring, collaborative practices, disease management, education, research, and administration. Key elements of cardiovascular nursing care at this level include the development, initiation, and maintenance of systems and processes that promote teamwork, collaboration, efficiency, and patient satisfaction.

Cardiovascular nursing research is a well-developed aspect of the cardiovascular nursing role. After years of research by nurses into the varied dimensions of practice described above as well as emerging areas like genomics, cardiovascular nursing research has broadened the scientific foundation of cardiovascular practice and provided evidence of effective approaches to cardiovascular nursing care.

The Evolution of Cardiovascular Nursing Practice

The first scope and standards for cardiovascular nursing were developed and published in 1975 in collaboration with the American Heart Association (AHA), and updated in 1981. Since that time the scope of practice of cardiovascular nursing has expanded dramatically, coinciding with the explosion of new evidence about cardiovascular disease epidemiology and pathophysiology across the lifespan, its assessment, diagnosis, treatment, and outcomes. (These predecessor publications are reproduced in Appendixes B, C, and D.)

The scope of practice initially included hospital-based care for individuals experiencing acute, chronic, and critical cardiovascular illnesses. It has since evolved to include prevention, risk modification, and care across the full spectrum of healthcare settings for those who are stable, those with medically unstable chronic cardiovascular illness, and those with major co-morbidities that affect cardiovascular illness assessment, diagnosis, treatment, and outcomes. The current practice of cardiovascular nursing requires extensive clinical knowledge and expertise to provide highly specialized acute, critical, or end-of-life care to hospitalized patients. The practice has also expanded to include an increased emphasis on prevention of cardiovascular disease, providing interventions and care in diverse settings including ambulatory and home-based venues. Cardiovascular nurses partner with patients, families, and other healthcare providers to enhance self-care utilizing innovative models of symptom and disease management in order to improve patient outcomes.

The greater complexity of cardiovascular disease creates crucial roles for cardiovascular nurses as caregivers, coordinators, educators, administrators, case managers, and quality specialists who optimize patient outcomes associated with specific cardiovascular diagnoses. Cardiovascular nurses provide multiple and complex treatments, many of which are initiated or led by nurses. For example, patient education and counseling may involve knowledge and skills in several cardiovascular subspecialities because many patients have numerous concurrent conditions such as hypertension, coronary artery disease, atrial fibrillation, and systolic heart failure. Thus, education must meet the self-care needs of patients with multiple medical conditions. The cardiovascular nurse must be sufficiently knowledgeable to teach patients and families about multiple topics such as diet, exercise or activity, medications, signs and symptoms of worsening condition, self-management behaviors when signs or symptoms emerge or worsen, when to notify a healthcare provider, the type of healthcare provider to call first, as well as medical and nursing research results, diagnostic testing, and new treatments.

Thus, a cardiovascular nurse seeks to go beyond a general nursing role of one who happens to be caring for patients with cardiovascular illnesses or working in a setting—in any capacity—focused on cardiovascular prevention. Rather, a cardiovascular nurse demonstrates a strong interest in the population, a quest for knowledge, and a desire to increase personal competence in the field. The term *cardiovascular nurse* connotes the expectation of a level of cardiovascular care knowledge (basic or advanced) and skills related to the care setting, that entails synthesis of incoming data, delivery of actions, and evaluation steps that ultimately help individuals or groups attain, maintain, or restore cardiovascular health, or meet a peaceful death.

Cardiovascular nurse roles include increasing levels of responsibility, including the development of advanced practice nursing roles such as clinical nurse specialists (CNSs) and nurse practitioners (NPs). More than a dozen professional organizations serve the educational and professional needs of cardiovascular nurses. This revised scope and standards for cardiovascular nursing document is unique in that it is a unifying effort to describe cardiovascular nursing practice based on the participation and contribution of 14 nursing organizations whose constituency includes cardiovascular nurses. (Summary descriptions and the websites of these organizations are in Appendix A.) This document will serve as a new foundation for cardiovascular nursing that will require ongoing assessment and evaluation, so that it consistently represents the state of the art for cardiovascular nursing practice.

Practice Characteristics

Cardiovascular care is collaborative in nature. Cardiovascular nurses partner with physicians and many other members of the healthcare team in a wide range of practice settings, including acute care, skilled nursing facilities, and home settings. An essential nursing role in these settings is direct or indirect contact with individuals with actual or potential cardiovascular disease. Cardiovascular nurses work at the bedside in acute care settings (emergency, perioperative, acute, progressive, and intensive care settings for children and adults), in transplant programs, in cardiac rehabilitation, in offices and clinics where cardiology or cardiovascular surgery is emphasized, and in community health, home care, and hospice or palliative care. Many cardiovascular nurses work in general practice settings such as family practice, pediatrics, obstetrics, internal medicine, and gerontology practices with large patient populations who are aging and at risk for or who have cardiovascular disease. Cardiovascular nurses work in other diverse settings such as telemonitoring, information technology, cardiac catheterization and electrophysiology laboratories, noninvasive imaging, radiology, exercise testing, heart failure clinics and transplantation programs, and the pharmaceutical and device industries.

Cardiovascular nurses also provide even more specialized cardiovascular care by managing and directing clinics focused on risk reduction, anticoagulation, lipid, hypertension, heart failure, cardiac rhythm management, life-sustaining and lifesaving devices, infusion therapies, genetics, peripartum care, and pediatric or adult congenital heart disease. Because nursing practice may be dictated by the patient population (e.g., pediatric, elderly, hypertension, heart failure) or setting (e.g., critical or ambulatory care), cardiovascular nurse training, professional development, and advanced specialized clinical knowledge and skills must be commensurate with the nursing practice needs of the patient population and setting.

Educational Requirements for General Cardiovascular Nurses

Cardiovascular nurses include licensed registered nurses and advanced practice nurses (nurse practitioners or clinical nurse specialists), nurse educators, administrators, case managers, quality specialists, and researchers. An RN, regardless of specialty, is licensed and authorized by a state, commonwealth, or territory to practice nursing. The RN is educationally prepared for competent practice at the beginning novice level upon graduating from an approved school of nursing and qualified national examination for RN licensure. Since 1965, the American Nurses

Association (ANA) has consistently affirmed the baccalaureate degree in nursing as the preferred educational preparation for entry into nursing practice. However, new nurses may enter the profession with diploma, associate, baccalaureate, generic master's, or doctoral degrees.

All RNs begin their education in the science and art of nursing with an overall goal of helping individuals or groups attain, maintain, and restore health whenever possible. Experienced nurses become proficient in one or more practice areas or roles, and may focus on patient care in clinical nursing practice specialties, such as cardiovascular nursing. Specialized cardiovascular knowledge and experience may be acknowledged through an identified certification process, in which specific nursing educational requirements and demonstration of knowledge in cardiovascular nursing practice have been delineated and validated (e.g., the ANCC and ACCN Cardiac/Vascular Nursing exams, or the CCRN Critical Care exam).

Registered nurses may elect to pursue studies for advanced cardiovascular nursing specialization. Educational requirements vary by specialty, role, and educational institution. Upon graduation, cardiovascular nurses may pursue national certification in a variety of direct and indirect care roles (e.g., adult health, critical care, community health, clinical nurse specialist, or nurse practitioner). In response to changing healthcare, education, and regulatory environments, models of education continue to evolve. Advanced practice certification examinations for cardiovascular nursing are currently being developed.

To provide general cardiovascular nursing care, nurses need a broad knowledge base in anatomy, physiology, pharmacology, pharmacogenomics, pharmacotherapeutics, nutrition, psychology, sociology, and developmental theory. The professional cardiovascular general practice nurse requires a specialty knowledge base, as indicated above. Clinical competencies beyond that obtained in basic nursing education include assessment and management of cardiovascular conditions, education and counseling skills for comprehensive cardiovascular risk factor reduction, disease management, and encouraging patients in a lifelong pattern of healthy living.

Competencies in addressing the physiological, psychosocial, educational, and spiritual needs of patients living with chronic cardiovascular illness are essential, including skill in helping patients and families deal with aging and end-of-life issues. Cardiovascular nurses must be knowledgeable of the principles of ethical practice and have resources available to evaluate the merits, risks, and social concerns of cardiovascular interventions. In addition, as part of autonomous cardiovascular nursing practice, nurses must be educated in patient advocacy across the age spectrum. Starting with nutritional support and avoidance of teratogens at conception, education on healthy nutrition and exercise is essential, along with garnering greater public support for the elderly because of their increased incidence of cardiovascular disease.

The core of cardiovascular nursing practice centers on the use of clinical judgment and decision-making based on scientific information and theory, and evidenced-based guidelines as they relate to cardiovascular care. In providing comprehensive care across the continuum from prevention to end of life, the general cardiovascular nurse uses the nursing process to assess individual and group needs, to form an appropriate nursing diagnosis, to design a mutually agreed upon plan of care, to coordinate and provide therapeutic interventions, to document the care, and to evaluate this action plan using a multidisciplinary case management approach.

Strong assessment skills are the foundation of cardiovascular nursing practice. These include both cardiac and vascular system assessment in addition to all affected systems. Intensive knowledge of cardiovascular physiology is necessary, including the principles of electrophysiology and dysrhythmia recognition, as these are required by all cardiovascular nurses to accurately assess and respond appropriately to life-threatening conditions.

With the explosion of knowledge has come complex equipment to evaluate, monitor, and treat cardiovascular patients. This equipment varies in complexity from simple diagnostic tools such as the stethoscope and sphygmomanometer, to complex imaging systems that can diagnose a congenital heart defect before 20 weeks gestational age, reconstruct damaged or defective hearts, and guide catheters into coronary arteries. Patient monitoring systems likewise have evolved from simple bedside monitors of electrocardiograms to implantable devices to document arrhythmias. With the development of small chip microprocessors, cardiac rhythm management devices have become extremely complex and can monitor hemodynamic changes, analyze cardiac rhythms, and provide therapy for potentially fatal arrhythmias. Mechanical circulatory support has evolved from bridge devices for cardiac transplantation to end-stage heart failure treatment for select patient populations. As a result, cardiovascular nurses require a general working knowledge of these aspects of care.

Many general cardiovascular nurses learn to use and monitor the data from catheters and devices associated with medical, surgical, and preventive care for all ages of people with cardiovascular conditions. Examples include pulmonary artery catheters, thoracic impedance or hemodynamic monitoring devices (internal or external systems), cardiac rhythm management devices, and mechanical circulatory support devices. With their expertise in these advanced technologies, cardiovascular nurses can assure patient safety during their use, monitor the function of and manage information provided by the equipment, assess patient responses, and teach patients and families about the temporary and long-term use of these devices.

A strong cardiovascular knowledge base is necessary for cardiovascular administrators, researchers, case managers, transplant coordinators, quality specialists, and educators in cardiovascular disease; they need a thorough preparation in their area of service in addition to nurse provider knowledge.

Advanced Practice Cardiovascular Nursing

Registered nurses with graduate education and advanced specialized clinical knowledge and skills are advanced practice registered nurses (APRNs), including clinical nurse specialists (CNSs) and nurse practitioners (NPs). APRNs have earned an advanced nursing degree and demonstrate a greater depth and breadth of nursing knowledge, synthesis of data, advanced nursing skills, and significant autonomy. Although the scope of practice for RNs and APRNs is distinctly different, there is an overlap in some cardiovascular knowledge and skills.

NPs specializing in cardiovascular care are registered nurses with a master's or doctoral degree as an nurse practitioner. The role requires expanded knowledge and skills for providing expert care to individuals, groups, or populations at risk for or diagnosed with cardiovascular disease. They conduct comprehensive assessments and promote health and prevention of cardiovascular injury and disease. A cardiovascular NP develops differential diagnoses, orders tests and procedures, performs physical examinations, interprets diagnostic and laboratory tests, makes a diagnosis, and prescribes pharmacologic and non-pharmacologic therapies for the direct management and treatment of acute and chronic cardiovascular illness and disease.

Cardiovascular NPs provide evidenced-based health and medical care in primary, acute, and long-term settings, and practice both autonomously and in collaboration with other healthcare professionals to treat and manage cardiovascular health problems. They promote cardiovascular health and disease prevention through patient and community education, advocating for heart-healthy life styles, performing cardiovascular risk assessment, and implementing risk factor modifications. Cardiovascular NPs serve in a variety of settings as researchers, consultants, and patient advocates to individuals, families, groups, and communities.

Cardiovascular CNSs are registered nurses who have graduate-level nursing preparation at the master's or doctoral degree level as a CNS. They are clinical experts in evidence-based cardiovascular nursing practice, treating and managing the health problems of cardiovascular patients and populations. Cardiovascular CNSs practice autonomously, integrating knowledge of disease and medical conditions into the assessment, diagnosis, and treatment of patients' cardiovascular illnesses. They also work collaboratively with other members of the healthcare team.

These nurses design, implement, and evaluate both patient-specific and population-based programs of care. Cardiovascular CNSs provide leadership in advancing the practice of cardiovascular nursing to achieve quality and cost-effective patient outcomes. They lead multidisciplinary groups in designing and implementing innovative alternative solutions that address systems and patient care issues. As direct care providers, cardiovascular CNSs perform comprehensive health assessments, develop differential diagnoses, and may have prescriptive authority, which allows them to prescribe pharmacologic and non-pharmacologic agents for the direct management and treatment of acute and chronic cardiovascular illness and disease. Cardiovascular CNSs serve as patient advocates and educators. They provide expert consultation and education to healthcare providers, and conduct and interpret research to improve practices and enhance patient outcomes.

Continuing Professional Development and Lifelong Learning

Cardiovascular nursing professional development is a lifelong process of active participation by the cardiovascular generalist or advanced practice registered nurse (APRN) in learning to acquire and maintain competence, enhance professional practice, and achieve career goals. Cardiovascular nursing professional development begins with the basic academic nursing preparation and continues throughout the professional life of the cardiovascular nurse.

Lifelong learning, which is the obligation and responsibility of all nurses, is expected and necessary to maintain and increase competency in cardiovascular nursing practice. Continuing competence is essential to the provision of safe, quality health care to cardiovascular patients and ensures that the nurse can perform in a changing healthcare environment. Continuing competence is the hallmark of professionalism and a means by which a professional is held accountable to society. Competence is reflected in the nurse's ability to use their knowledge, skill, judgment, abilities, values, and beliefs to deliver quality care to cardiovascular patients in a variety of situations and practice settings. All cardiovascular patients are entitled to receive care from cardiovascular nurses who maintain professional nursing competence.

Cardiovascular nursing professional development encompasses the domains of academic education, continuing education, and staff development. Academic education consists of courses taken for credit in an institution of higher education that may or may not lead to a degree, completion of a certification program, or individual coursework taken to update oneself in the cardiovascular specialty. Continuing education comprises a systematic professional learning experience designed to augment the knowledge, skills, and abilities, thereby enriching the nurse's contribution to quality health care. Continuing education can be part of a formal academic program, part of staff development, or studying for the purpose of enhancing cardiovascular nursing practice. Staff development is the systematic process of assessment, planning, education, and evaluation that enhances the performance or professional growth of the nurse. Staff development can include continuing education and academic education.

Specialty Certification

Certification in the United States is a voluntary process whereby a nongovernmental agency, such as the American Nurses Credentialing Center (ANCC), the American Association of Critical-Care Nurses Credentialing Center, or another professional organization, recognizes and validates an individual's knowledge, skills, and abilities in a defined area of nursing practice. This professional certification represents the recognition of the excellence and continued competency of the nurse and serves to assure the public of competent professional practice. Certification is accomplished by meeting pre-established standards, usually including the successful completion of an examination.

Nurses who achieve certification in cardiovascular nursing assure clients, patients, and families that they possess the knowledge and skills needed to give excellent cardiovascular care. Cardiovascular nursing examinations incorporate the domains of practice described above. Some cardiovascular nurses may choose to attain interdisciplinary certifications which demonstrate expertise in use of specific technologies (e.g., interrogation and reprogramming of permanent pacemakers) or skills (e.g., clinical management of organ transplant recipients, health-care quality management). Advanced practice certification examinations for cardiovascular nursing are not available at this time, but are currently being developed.

Future Considerations

A host of issues and trends in health care influence specialty nursing care for individuals and families at risk for or with cardiovascular health problems. As the baby boomers age, the sheer volume of people requiring cardiovascular care will have a significant impact on healthcare resources and demands for services through 2020, and will directly affect the cardiovascular nursing profession. New discoveries about the genetic and pathophysiologic origins of disease and how they interact with environment and lifestyle have added to our already vast knowledge, challenging those in the nursing profession to stay well-informed for their roles in providing care, advocating for patient needs, and teaching patients and their families. Emerging science about novel risk factors that increase the probability of cardiovascular disease, new diagnostic tests and treatments, and advances in genomics and genetics, including pharmacogenomics, will shape treatment choices in the future. Cardiovascular nurses are challenged to engage in lifelong learning in order to keep abreast of the rapidly developing science and to always provide evidence-based nursing care. The translation of new knowledge and evidence must be accelerated.

The explosion of new information has heightened the importance of the use of evidence in providing care and counseling for patients about their therapeutic options. Thus, maintaining current knowledge in this era of evidence-based practice is both challenging and essential. A variety of issues related to the current nursing workforce and work environments warrant attention in planning for future cardiovascular health care. The continuing shortage of nurses, aggravated by the aging nursing workforce, is well-documented. Work environments for nurses must be transformed in order to retain experienced practitioners. Nurses must be involved in decisions related to creating patient care systems and healthy work environments. Continued efforts and funding to support nursing education are also essential to ensure adequate numbers of knowledgeable and competent cardiovascular nurses. New specialized healthcare provider roles increase the risk of fragmented, discontinuous care and poor communication. Enhanced skills in interdisciplinary communication and collaboration will be required of nurses in order to ensure patient safety and coordination of care.

Projected shortages of primary care physicians and changes in medical education provide opportunities for advanced practice nurses but deplete the number of nurses available at the bedside. At the same time, physician shortages provide an opportunity for advanced practice nurses to collaborate with physicians, registered nurses, and healthcare executives to reconfigure care systems and develop structures and processes that promote evidence-based practice. Advanced practice nurses are also integral to efforts to improve interdisciplinary communication, interpret and accelerate the application of evidence to patient care, conduct research, and improve outcomes of care.

Issues specific to care environments include technology, work force, safety, and patient transitions. As the rate of technological advances increases, cardiovascular nurses need to be competent in the application and evaluation of technology, which incorporates ethical decisions in the use of the technology. The incidence of adverse events and medical errors in all healthcare settings mandates a continued emphasis on safety and quality initiatives in caring for patients with cardiovascular healthcare needs.

Fragmentation of care contributes to a greater need for nurses to be able to provide seamless care and excellent communication as patients move between acute care and community or home settings. The shift of hospital-based therapies to ambulatory and home care settings requires a competent and knowledgeable nursing workforce, regardless of the setting where patients receive care. Telehealth technologies, which help nurses to assess, monitor, and treat patients remotely, require technological expertise, knowledge of transitional care issues, and vigilance to ensure continuing communication with patients and families about their nursing care needs.

The growing number of infants and elderly patients with complex cardiovascular disease complicated by comorbidities, combined with shortened hospital stays, will require cardiovascular nurses to address the complexities involved in the transition of patients from hospital to home or long-term care or its future alternatives. Increased communication between ambulatory and home-based care providers, improved discharge planning, and better training of families and caregivers to manage illness and appropriately access the healthcare system are needed.

The complexity of the healthcare system remains a challenge for many patients and families who desire a more active role in decision-making about health. Self-care and increased healthcare consumerism provide nurses with unique opportunities to influence outcomes. Quality of life, and how it affects patients' decisions about new therapies, is an important consideration, as are the knowledge, skills, and emotions of the family or caregiver. Advances in science, and patient longevity, afford nurses even greater opportunity to influence target audiences at multiple points across the life span. Emphasis on the patient's personal responsibility for improving health can foster stronger partnerships with healthcare decision-makers considering various treatment options.

Initiatives in health promotion and disease prevention continue to be under-funded by insurance companies in most healthcare systems. The need to justify costly health care with improved outcomes has renewed the focus on prevention. However, standardized coding systems downplay interdisciplinary efforts, resulting in decreased reimbursement for such efforts and limiting innovation to meet these goals. Increasing financial burdens on consumers, employers, and government resources are providing opportunities for nurses to become part of future solutions. Given the prevalence of people who are living with chronic, preventable cardiovascular conditions, cardiovascular nurses are in a unique position to create programs for individuals and communities.

Preventing cardiovascular disease starts in infancy. Helping people avoid obesity, stop smoking, be more active, and eat better can significantly reduce morbidity and mortality associated with cardiovascular disease. Cardiovascular nurses will need to apply emerging knowledge of how successful behavioral change happens if they are to lead patients to adopt healthier lifestyles.

The healthcare needs of underserved and ethnically diverse populations provide both opportunities and responsibilities for nurses. Advanced practice nurses with expertise in physiology, medicine, and behavioral change contribute to improvements in the health of patients and families. Cardiovascular nurses bring unique knowledge, skills, and expertise that can be used to create innovative programs for improving the health of patients, families, and communities. Together, this competent and caring nursing workforce has the knowledge and expertise needed to care for the nearly 80 million people who are living with cardiovascular disease in the United States.

This current scope and standards for cardiovascular nursing will of necessity be a living document, continually updated as our understanding and management of cardiovascular disease advances. In its current form it should provide the foundation for sound cardiovascular nursing practice.

Additional Content

For a better appreciation of the historical and professional context underlying the publication of *Cardiovascular Nursing: Scope and Standards of Practice*, the contents of three predecessor publications—the successive 1975 and 1981 editions of the standards of cardiovascular nursing practice, along with the related 1993 scope of cardiac rehabilitation practice—have been included in the text and indexed with the current content of this edition.

- Appendix B: *The Scope of Cardiac Rehabilitation Practice* (1993)
- Appendix C: *Standards of Cardiovascular Nursing Practice* (1981)
- Appendix D: *Standards of Cardiovascular Nursing Practice* (1975)

STANDARDS OF CARDIOVASCULAR NURSING PRACTICE

STANDARDS OF PRACTICE

STANDARD 1. ASSESSMENT
The cardiovascular registered nurse collects comprehensive data pertinent to the patient's health or the situation.

Measurement Criteria:

The cardiovascular registered nurse:

- Collects data in a systematic and ongoing process.

- Involves the patient, family, other healthcare providers, and environment as appropriate in holistic data collection.

- Is involved in assessment of patients of all ages across the continuum of care from acute to community care.

- Prioritizes data collection activities based on the patient's immediate condition, or anticipated needs of the patient or situation.

- Uses developmentally appropriate evidence-based assessment techniques and instruments in collecting pertinent data.

- Uses analytical models and problem-solving tools.

- Synthesizes available data, information, and knowledge relevant to the situation to identify patterns and variances.

- Documents relevant data in a retrievable format.

Additional Measurement Criteria for the Advanced Practice Registered Nurse:

The advanced practice cardiovascular registered nurse:

- Initiates and interprets diagnostic tests and procedures relevant to the patient's current status.

STANDARD 2. DIAGNOSIS
The cardiovascular registered nurse analyzes the assessment data to determine the nursing diagnoses or health-related issues.

Measurement Criteria:

The cardiovascular registered nurse:

- Derives the diagnoses or issues based on assessment data that reflect the patient's current clinical condition.

- Systematically compares and contrasts clinical findings with normal and abnormal variations.

- Derives diagnoses encompassing:
  - The patient's identified or potential physiological, psychological, and developmental problems.
  - The needs of the child or adolescent to attend school.
  - The needs of the elderly patient regarding integration into post-hospital or long-term care.
  - The support and educational needs of the family or designated care provider.
  - Any present or potential environmental problems.

- Refines and revises diagnoses regularly, based on data subsequently collected.

- Discusses diagnoses and cardiovascular risk factors with the patient, family, caregivers, members of the interdisciplinary team, and other healthcare providers when possible and appropriate.

- Documents diagnoses or issues in a manner that facilitates the determination of the expected outcomes and plan.

Additional Measurement Criteria for the Advanced Practice Registered Nurse:

The advanced practice cardiovascular registered nurse:

- Systematically compares and contrasts clinical findings with normal and abnormal variations and developmental events in formulating a differential diagnosis.

- Utilizes complex data and information obtained during interview, examination, and diagnostic procedures in identifying diagnoses.

- Assists staff in developing and maintaining competency in the diagnostic process.

STANDARD 3. OUTCOMES IDENTIFICATION
The cardiovascular registered nurse identifies expected outcomes for a plan individualized to the patient or the situation.

Measurement Criteria:

The cardiovascular registered nurse:

- Identifies expected outcomes mutually with the patient, family, and other healthcare providers. Expected outcomes are patient-oriented, developmentally appropriate, evidenced-based, and attainable given the patient's and family's present and potential capabilities.

- Derives culturally and age-appropriate expected outcomes from the diagnoses.

- Considers associated risks, benefits, costs, current scientific evidence, and clinical expertise when formulating expected outcomes.

- Defines expected outcomes in terms of the patient, patient values, ethical considerations, environment, or situation with such consideration as associated risks, benefits and costs, and current scientific evidence.

- Includes a time estimate for attainment of expected outcomes.

- Develops expected outcomes that provide direction for continuity of care.

- Modifies expected outcomes based on changes in the status of the patient or evaluation of the situation.

- Documents expected outcomes as measurable goals.

- Implements national consensus-based clinical guidelines.

Additional Measurement Criteria for the Advanced Practice Registered Nurse:

The advanced practice cardiovascular registered nurse:

- Identifies expected outcomes that incorporate scientific evidence and are achievable through implementation of evidence-based practices.

- Identifies expected outcomes that incorporate cost and clinical effectiveness, patient satisfaction, and continuity and consistency among providers.

- Supports the use of clinical guidelines linked to positive patient outcomes.

STANDARD 4. PLANNING

The cardiovascular registered nurse develops a plan that prescribes strategies and alternatives to attain expected outcomes.

Measurement Criteria:

The cardiovascular registered nurse:

- Develops an individualized cardiovascular plan considering patient characteristics, developmental level, and situation (e.g., age- and culturally appropriate, environmentally sensitive).

- Participates in the design and development of multidisciplinary and interdisciplinary processes to address the situation or issue.

- Contributes to the development and continuous improvement of organizational systems that support the planning process.

- Supports the integration of clinical, human, and financial resources to enhance and complete the decision-making processes.

- Develops the plan in conjunction with the patient, family, and others, synthesizing patients' values and beliefs, developmental level, and coping style.

- Includes strategies in the plan that address each of the identified diagnoses or issues, which may include strategies for promotion and restoration of health and prevention of illness, injury, and disease.

- Provides for continuity in the plan.

- Incorporates an implementation pathway or timeline in the plan.

- Establishes the plan priorities with the patient, family, and others as appropriate.

- Utilizes the plan to provide direction to other members of the healthcare team.

- Defines the plan to reflect current statutes, rules and regulations, and standards of cardiovascular nursing practice.

- Integrates current trends and research affecting care in the planning process.

- Considers the economic impact of the plan for the patient, family, caregivers, or other affected parties.

- Uses standardized language or recognized terminology to document the plan.

Additional Measurement Criteria for the Advanced Practice Registered Nurse:

The advanced practice cardiovascular registered nurse:

- Identifies assessment, diagnostic strategies, and therapeutic interventions in the plan that reflect current evidence, including data, research, literature, and expert clinical knowledge.

- Selects or designs strategies to meet the multifaceted needs of complex patients.

- Includes the synthesis of patients' values and beliefs regarding nursing and medical therapies in the plan.

STANDARD 5. IMPLEMENTATION
The cardiovascular registered nurse implements the identified plan.

Measurement Criteria:

The cardiovascular registered nurse:

- Implements the plan in a safe and timely manner.

- Implements the plan using principles and concepts of project or systems management.

- Fosters organizational systems that support implementation of the plan.

- Documents implementation and any modifications, including changes or omissions, of the identified plan.

- Utilizes evidence-based interventions and treatments specific to the diagnosis or problem.

- Facilitates utilization of systems and community resources to implement the plan.

- Collaborates with nursing colleagues and other disciplines to implement the plan.

- Incorporates new knowledge and strategies to initiate change in nursing care practices if desired outcomes are not achieved.

Additional Measurement Criteria for the Advanced Practice Registered Nurse:

The advanced practice cardiovascular registered nurse:

- Facilitates utilization of systems and community resources to implement the plan.

- Supports collaboration with nursing colleagues and other disciplines to implement the plan.

- Incorporates new knowledge and strategies to initiate change in nursing care practices if desired outcomes are not achieved.

STANDARD 5A. COORDINATION OF CARE
The cardiovascular registered nurse coordinates care delivery.

Measurement Criteria:

The cardiovascular registered nurse:

- Provides leadership in the coordination of multidisciplinary health care for integrated delivery of patient care services.
- Documents the coordination of care.
- Synthesizes data and information to facilitate necessary system and community support measures, including environmental modifications.
- Coordinates system and community resources that enhance delivery of care across the continuum.

Measurement Criteria for the Advanced Practice Registered Nurse:

The advanced practice cardiovascular registered nurse:

- Provides leadership in the coordination of multidisciplinary health care for integrated delivery of patient care services.
- Synthesizes data and information to prescribe necessary system and community support measures, including environmental modifications.
- Coordinates system and community resources that enhance delivery of care across continuums.

STANDARD 5B. HEALTH TEACHING AND HEALTH PROMOTION
The cardiovascular registered nurse employs strategies to promote health and a safe environment.

Measurement Criteria:

The cardiovascular registered nurse:

- Provides health teaching that addresses such topics as healthy lifestyles, risk-reducing behaviors, developmental needs, activities of daily living, and preventive self-care.

- Uses health promotion and health teaching methods appropriate to the situation and the patient's developmental level, learning needs, readiness, ability to learn, literacy level, language preference, and culture.

- Seeks opportunities for feedback and evaluation of the effectiveness of the strategies used.

Additional Measurement Criteria for the Advanced Practice Registered Nurse:

The advanced practice cardiovascular registered nurse:

- Synthesizes empirical evidence on risk behaviors, learning theories, behavioral change theories, motivational theories, epidemiology, and other related theories and frameworks when designing health information and patient education.

- Designs health information and patient education appropriate to the patient's developmental level, learning needs, readiness to learn, and cultural values and beliefs.

- Evaluates health information resources, such as Internet sites, within the area of practice for accuracy, readability, and comprehensibility to help patients access quality health information.

STANDARD 5C. CONSULTATION

The cardiovascular registered nurse provides consultation to influence the identified plan, enhance the abilities of others, and effect change.

Measurement Criteria:

The cardiovascular registered nurse:

- Synthesizes clinical data, theoretical frameworks, and evidence when providing consultation.

- Facilitates the effectiveness of a consultation by involving the patient and family in decision-making and negotiating role responsibilities.

- Communicates consultation recommendations to facilitate change.

- Communicates consultation recommendations that influence the identified plan, facilitates understanding by involved stakeholders, enhances the work of others, and effects change.

Additional Measurement Criteria for the Advanced Practice Registered Nurse:

The advanced practice cardiovascular registered nurse:

- Synthesizes complex clinical data, theoretical frameworks, and evidence when providing consultation.

- Facilitates the effectiveness of a consultation by involving the patient and family in decision-making and negotiating role responsibilities.

- Facilitates the effectiveness of a consultation by conducting research and disseminating research findings to enhance interaction meaningfulness (psychosocial or clinical outcomes).

- Directs consultation recommendations that facilitate change.

STANDARD 5D. PRESCRIPTIVE AUTHORITY AND TREATMENT

The advanced practice cardiovascular registered nurse uses prescriptive authority, procedures, referrals, treatments, and therapies in accordance with state and federal laws and regulations.

Measurement Criteria for the Advanced Practice Registered Nurse:

The advanced practice cardiovascular registered nurse:

- Prescribes evidence-based treatments, therapies, and procedures considering the patient's comprehensive healthcare needs.

- Prescribes pharmacologic agents based on a current knowledge of pharmacology and physiology.

- Prescribes specific pharmacological agents or treatments based on clinical indicators, the patient's status and needs, and the results of diagnostic and laboratory tests.

- Evaluates therapeutic and potential adverse effects of pharmacological and non-pharmacological treatments.

- Provides patients with information about intended effects and potential adverse effects of proposed prescriptive therapies.

- Provides information about costs, and alternative treatments and procedures, as appropriate.

STANDARD 6. EVALUATION
The cardiovascular registered nurse evaluates progress towards attainment of outcomes.

Measurement Criteria:

The cardiovascular registered nurse:

- Conducts a systematic, ongoing, and criterion-based evaluation of the outcomes in relation to the structures and processes prescribed by the plan and the indicated timeline.

- Includes the patient and others involved in the care or situation in the evaluative process.

- Evaluates the effectiveness of the planned strategies in relation to patient responses and the attainment of the expected outcomes.

- Documents the results of the evaluation.

- Uses ongoing assessment data to revise the diagnoses, the outcomes, the plan, and the implementation as needed.

- Disseminates the results to the patient and others involved in the care or situation, as appropriate, in accordance with state and federal laws and regulations.

Additional Measurement Criteria for the Advanced Practice Registered Nurse:

The advanced practice cardiovascular registered nurse:

- Evaluates the accuracy of the diagnosis and effectiveness of the interventions in relationship to the patient's attainment of expected outcomes.

- Synthesizes the results of the evaluation to determine the impact of the plan on the affected patients, families, groups, communities, and institutions.

- Uses the results of the evaluation to make or recommend process or structural changes including policy, procedure, or protocol documentation, as appropriate.

STANDARDS OF PROFESSIONAL PERFORMANCE

STANDARD 7. QUALITY OF PRACTICE
The cardiovascular registered nurse systematically enhances the quality and effectiveness of nursing practice.

Measurement Criteria:

The cardiovascular registered nurse:

- Demonstrates quality by documenting the application of the nursing process in a responsible, accountable, and ethical manner.

- Uses the results of quality improvement activities to initiate changes in nursing practice and in the healthcare delivery system.

- Uses creativity and innovation in nursing practice to improve care delivery.

- Incorporates new knowledge to initiate changes in nursing practice if desired outcomes are not achieved.

- Obtains and maintains professional certification if available in the area of expertise.

- Designs and participates in quality improvement activities. Such activities may include:

  - Identifying aspects of practice important for quality monitoring.

  - Using indicators developed to monitor quality and effectiveness of nursing practice.

  - Collecting data to monitor quality and effectiveness of nursing practice.

  - Analyzing quality data to identify opportunities for improving nursing practice.

  - Formulating recommendations to improve nursing practice or outcomes.

  - Implementing activities to enhance the quality of nursing practice.

Continued ▶

- Developing, implementing, and evaluating policies, procedures, and guidelines to improve the quality of practice.

- Participating on interdisciplinary teams to evaluate clinical care or health services.

- Participating in efforts to minimize costs and unnecessary duplication.

- Analyzing factors related to safety, satisfaction, effectiveness, and cost–benefit options.

- Analyzing organizational systems for barriers.

- Implementing processes to remove or decrease barriers within organizational systems.

Additional Measurement Criteria for the Advanced Practice Registered Nurse:

The advanced practice cardiovascular registered nurse:

- Obtains and maintains professional certification if available in the area of expertise.

- Designs quality improvement initiatives.

- Implements initiatives to evaluate the need for change.

- Evaluates the practice environment and quality of nursing care in relation to existing evidence, identifying opportunities for the generation and use of research.

STANDARD 8. EDUCATION

The cardiovascular registered nurse attains knowledge and competency that reflects current nursing practice.

Measurement Criteria:

The cardiovascular registered nurse:

- Participates in ongoing educational activities related to appropriate knowledge bases and professional issues.

- Demonstrates a commitment to lifelong learning through self-reflection and inquiry to identify learning needs.

- Seeks experiences that reflect current practice in order to maintain skills and competence in clinical practice or role performance.

- Acquires knowledge and skills appropriate to the specialty area, practice setting, role, or situation.

- Maintains professional records that provide evidence of competency and lifelong learning.

- Seeks experiences and formal and independent learning activities to maintain and develop clinical and professional skills and knowledge.

- Obtains and maintains professional certification if available in the area of expertise.

Additional Measurement Criteria for the Advanced Practice Registered Nurse:

The advanced practice cardiovascular registered nurse:

- Uses current healthcare research findings and other evidence to expand clinical knowledge, enhance role performance, and increase knowledge of professional issues.

STANDARD 9. PROFESSIONAL PRACTICE EVALUATION

The cardiovascular registered nurse evaluates one's own nursing practice in relation to professional practice standards and guidelines, relevant statutes, rules, and regulations.

Measurement Criteria:

The cardiovascular registered nurse:

- Applies knowledge of current practice standards, guidelines, statutes, rules, and regulations in practice.

- Provides age- and developmentally appropriate care in a culturally and ethnically sensitive manner.

- Engages in self-evaluation of practice on a regular basis, identifying areas of strength as well as areas in which professional development would be beneficial.

- Obtains informal feedback regarding one's own practice from patients, peers, professional colleagues, and others.

- Participates in systematic peer review as appropriate.

- Takes action to achieve goals identified during the evaluation process.

- Provides rationales for practice beliefs, decisions, and actions as part of the informal and formal evaluation processes.

Additional Measurement Criteria for the Advanced Practice Registered Nurse:

The advanced practice cardiovascular registered nurse:

- Engages in a formal process seeking feedback regarding one's own practice from patients, peers, professional colleagues, and others.

STANDARD 10. COLLEGIALITY

The cardiovascular registered nurse interacts with, and contributes to the professional development of, peers and colleagues.

Measurement Criteria:

The cardiovascular registered nurse:

- Shares knowledge and skills with peers and colleagues as evidenced by such activities as patient care conferences or presentations at formal or informal meetings.

- Mentors other registered nurses and colleagues as appropriate.

- Provides peers with feedback regarding their practice and role performance.

- Interacts with peers and colleagues to enhance one's own professional nursing practice and role performance.

- Actively participates in multidisciplinary teams that contribute to role development and nursing practice.

- Maintains compassionate and caring relationships with peers and colleagues.

- Contributes to an environment that is conducive to the education of healthcare professionals.

- Contributes to a supportive and healthy work environment.

Additional Measurement Criteria for the Advanced Practice Registered Nurse:

The advanced practice cardiovascular registered nurse:

- Models expert practice to multidisciplinary team members and healthcare consumers.

- Mentors other registered nurses and colleagues as appropriate.

- Participates in multidisciplinary teams that contribute to role development and advanced nursing practice and health care.

STANDARD 11. COLLABORATION

The cardiovascular registered nurse collaborates with the patient, the family, and others in the conduct of nursing practice.

Measurement Criteria:

The cardiovascular registered nurse:

- Communicates with patient, family, and healthcare providers regarding patient care and the nurse's role in the provision of that care.

- Collaborates in creating a documented plan focused on outcomes and decisions related to care and delivery of services that indicates communication with patients, families, and others.

- Consults with other disciplines to enhance patient care through multidisciplinary activities such as education, consultation, management, technological development, or research opportunities.

- Partners with others to effect change and generate positive outcomes through knowledge of the patient or situation.

- Documents referrals, including provisions for continuity of care.

Additional Measurement Criteria for the Advanced Practice Registered Nurse:

The advanced practice cardiovascular registered nurse:

- Partners with other disciplines to enhance patient care through interdisciplinary activities such as education, consultation, management, technological development, or research opportunities.

- Facilitates a multidisciplinary process with other members of the healthcare team.

- Documents plan of care communications, rationales for plan of care changes, and collaborative discussions to improve patient care.

Standard 12. Ethics

The cardiovascular registered nurse integrates ethical provisions into all areas of practice.

Measurement Criteria:

The cardiovascular registered nurse:

- Uses *Code of Ethics for Nurses with Interpretive Statements* (ANA 2001) to guide practice.

- Delivers care in a manner that preserves and protects patient autonomy, dignity, and rights.

- Maintains patient confidentiality within legal and regulatory parameters.

- Serves as a patient advocate assisting patients in developing skills for self-advocacy.

- Maintains a therapeutic and professional patient–nurse relationship within appropriate professional role boundaries.

- Demonstrates a commitment to practicing self-care, managing stress, and connecting with self and others.

- Contributes to resolving ethical issues of patients, colleagues, or systems as evidenced in such activities as participating on ethics committees.

- Reports illegal, incompetent, or impaired practices.

Additional Measurement Criteria for the Advanced Practice Registered Nurse:

The advanced practice cardiovascular registered nurse:

- Informs patients of the risks, benefits, and outcomes of healthcare regimens.

- Participates in interdisciplinary teams that address ethical risks, benefits, and outcomes.

- Develops or facilitates nursing research related to ethical issues that emerge during patient care experiences.

STANDARD 13. RESEARCH
The cardiovascular registered nurse integrates research findings into practice.

Measurement Criteria:

The cardiovascular registered nurse:

- Utilizes the best available evidence, including research findings, to guide practice decisions.

- Actively participates in research activities at various levels appropriate to the nurse's level of education and position. Such activities may include:

  - Identifying clinical problems specific to nursing research (patient care and nursing practice).

  - Participating in data collection (surveys, pilot projects, and formal studies).

  - Participating in a formal committee or program.

  - Sharing research or findings with peers and others.

  - Conducting research.

  - Critically analyzing and interpreting research for application to practice.

  - Using research findings in the development of policies, procedures, and standards of practice in patient care.

  - Incorporating research as a basis for learning.

Additional Measurement Criteria for the Advanced Practice Registered Nurse:

The advanced practice cardiovascular registered nurse:

- Contributes to nursing knowledge by conducting or synthesizing research that discovers, examines, and evaluates knowledge, theories, criteria, and creative approaches to improve healthcare practice.

- Formally disseminates research findings through activities such as presentations, publications, consultation, and journal clubs.

- Encourages and facilitates nursing research of cardiovascular care topics by mentoring the registered nurse.

STANDARD 14. RESOURCE UTILIZATION
The cardiovascular registered nurse considers factors related to safety, effectiveness, cost, and impact on practice in the planning and delivery of nursing services.

Measurement Criteria:

The cardiovascular registered nurse:

- Utilizes organizational and community resources to formulate multidisciplinary or interdisciplinary plans of care.

- Evaluates factors such as safety, effectiveness, availability, cost and benefits, efficiencies, and impact on practice when choosing among practice options that would result in the same expected outcome.

- Assists the patient and family in identifying and securing appropriate and available services to address health-related needs.

- Assigns or delegates tasks, based on the needs and condition of the patient, potential for harm, stability of the patient's condition, complexity of the task, and predictability of the outcome.

- Promotes activities that assist the patient and family in becoming informed consumers about the options, costs, risks, and benefits of treatment and care.

- Develops evaluation strategies to demonstrate cost effectiveness, cost-benefit, and efficiency factors associated with excellence in nursing practice.

Additional Measurement Criteria for the Advanced Practice Registered Nurse:

The advanced practice cardiovascular registered nurse:

- Utilizes organizational and community resources to formulate multidisciplinary or interdisciplinary plans of care.

- Develops innovative solutions for patient care problems that address effective resource utilization and maintenance of quality.

- Develops evaluation strategies to demonstrate cost effectiveness, cost benefit, and efficiency factors associated with nursing practice.

STANDARD 15. LEADERSHIP
The cardiovascular registered nurse provides leadership in the professional practice setting and the profession.

Measurement Criteria:

The cardiovascular registered nurse:

- Works to influence decision-making bodies to improve patient care.

- Engages in teamwork as a team player and a team builder.

- Works to create and maintain healthy work environments in local, regional, national, or international communities.

- Displays the ability to define a clear vision, the associated goals, and a plan to implement and measure progress.

- Demonstrates a commitment to continuous, lifelong learning for self and others.

- Teaches others to succeed by mentoring and other strategies.

- Exhibits creativity and flexibility through times of change.

- Demonstrates energy, excitement, and a passion for quality work.

- Willingly accepts mistakes by self and others, thereby creating a culture in which risk-taking is not only safe, but expected.

- Inspires loyalty through valuing of people as the most precious asset in an organization.

- Directs the coordination of care across settings and among caregivers, including oversight of licensed and unlicensed personnel in any assigned or delegated tasks.

- Serves in key roles in the work setting by participating in committees, councils, and administrative teams.

- Promotes advancement of the profession through participation in professional organizations.

Additional Measurement Criteria for the Advanced Practice Registered Nurse:
The advanced practice cardiovascular registered nurse:

- Works to influence decision-making bodies to improve patient care.
- Provides direction to enhance the effectiveness of the healthcare team.
- Initiates and revises protocols or guidelines to reflect evidence-based practice, to reflect accepted changes in care management, or to address emerging problems.
- Promotes communication of information and advancement of the profession through writing, publishing, and presentations for professional or lay audiences.
- Designs innovations to effect change in practice and improve health outcomes.

GLOSSARY

Adherence. See *Treatment Adherence.*

Assessment. The process by which the nurse, through interaction with the patient, significant others, and healthcare providers, collects and analyzes data about the patient. Data may include the following dimensions: physical, psychological, sociocultural, spiritual, cognitive, functional abilities, developmental, economic, and life-style.

Cardiovascular nursing. Specialized nursing care focused on the optimization of cardiovascular health across the lifespan from conception to death.

Caregiver. A person who provides direct care for another, such as a child, a dependent adult, the disabled, or the chronically ill.

Code of ethics. A list of provisions that makes explicit the primary goals, values, and obligations of the profession.

Continuity of care. An interdisciplinary process that includes patients and significant others in the development of a coordinated plan of care. This process facilitates the patient's transition between settings, based on changing needs and available resources.

Criteria. Relevant, measurable indicators of the standards of clinical nursing practice.

Data. Discrete entities that are described objectively without interpretation.

Diagnosis. A clinical judgment about the patient's response to actual or potential health conditions or needs. The diagnosis provides the basis for determination of a plan of care to achieve expected outcomes. Cardiovascular registered nurses utilize nursing or medical diagnoses depending upon educational and clinical preparation and legal authority.

Disease. A biological or psychosocial disorder of structure or function in a patient, especially one that produces specific signs or symptoms or that affects a specific part of the body, mind, or spirit.

Disease management. A coordinated healthcare process to improve the health status of a defined patient population over the entire course of the disease. Both disease care and prevention efforts are included along with initiatives to reduce healthcare costs by providing symptom management. Cardiovascular advanced practice registered nurses collaborate in providing disease management care along with other healthcare providers.

Environment. The atmosphere, milieu, or conditions in which an individual lives, works, or regularly spends significant time.

Evaluation. The process of determining both the patient's progress toward the attainment of expected outcomes and the effectiveness of nursing care.

Expected outcomes. End results that are measurable, desirable, and observable, and translate into observational behaviors.

Evidence-based practice. Health care founded on the collection, interpretation, and integration of valid, important, and applicable patient-reported, clinician-observed, or research-derived evidence. The best available evidence, moderated by patient circumstances and preferences, is applied to improve the quality of clinical judgments.

Family. Family of origin or significant others as identified by the patient.

Guidelines. Systematically developed statements based on available scientific evidence and expert opinion and an aspect of patient care management with the potential of improving the quality of clinical and consumer decision-making.

Health. An experience that is often expressed in terms of wellness and illness, and may occur in the presence or absence of disease or injury.

Healthcare provider. A person with special expertise who provides healthcare services or assistance to patients. This may include nurses, physicians, psychologists, social workers, nutritionists/dieticians, and various therapists.

Holistic. Based on an understanding that the patient is an interconnected entity and that physical, mental, social, and spiritual factors need to be included in any interventions.

Illness. The subjective experience of discomfort.

Implementation. Activities such as teaching, monitoring, providing, counseling, delegating, and coordinating. The patient, significant others, or healthcare providers maybe designated to implement interventions within the plan of care.

Information. Data that are interpreted, organized, or structured.

Interdisciplinary. Reliant on the overlapping skills and knowledge of each team member and discipline, resulting in synergistic effects where outcomes are enhanced and more comprehensive than the simple aggregation of the individual efforts.

Knowledge. Information that is synthesized so that relationships are identified and formalized.

Multidisciplinary. Reliant on each team member or discipline contributing discipline-specific skills.

Nurse. An individual who is licensed by a state agency to practice as a registered nurse.

Nursing. The diagnosis and treatment of human responses to actual or potential health behaviors.

Outcomes. Measurable, expected, patient-oriented goals that translate into observable behaviors.

Patient. Recipient of nursing care. The term *patient* is used to provide consistency and brevity, bearing in mind that the terms such as *patient, individual, family, group, community, or population,* may be better choices in some instances. When the patient is an individual, the focus is on the health state, problems, or needs of the individual. When the patient is a family or group, the focus is on the health state of the unit as a whole or the reciprocal effects of an individual's health state on the other members of the unit. When the patient is a community or population, the focus is on personal and environmental health and the health risks of the community or population.

Peer review. A collegial, systematic, and periodic process by which registered nurses are held accountable for practice and which fosters the refinement of knowledge, skills, and decision-making at all levels and in all areas of practice.

Plan. A comprehensive outline of the steps that need to be undertaken to attain expected outcomes.

Quality of care. The degree to which health services for patients, families, groups, communities, and populations increase the likelihood of desired health outcomes, and are consistent with current professional knowledge.

Quality of life. A person's general perception of happiness and satisfaction with life, which may include health, physical, psychological, financial, social, family, economic, and spiritual areas. Patients with cardiovascular disease may focus on health-related quality of life, a subcomponent of quality of life, which looks at the perception of how one's functioning is impacted by disease or illness.

Recipient of nursing care. A patient, group, family, community, or population.

Self-care maintenance. Treatment adherence, monitoring, and behaviors used by patients to maintain their health.

Self-care management. The decision-making process that patients use to manage symptoms.

Situation. A set of circumstances, conditions, or events.

Standard. An authoritative statement enunciated and promulgated by the profession, by which the quality of practice, service, or education can be judged.

Standards of nursing care. Authoritative statements that describe a level of care or performance common to the profession of nursing by which the quality of nursing practice can be judged. They include both standards of practice and standards of professional performance.

Standards of practice. Authoritative statements that describe a competent level of clinical nursing practice demonstrated through assessment, diagnosis, outcomes identification, planning, implementation, and evaluation.

Standards of professional performance. Authoritative statements that describe a competent level of behavior in the professional role, including activities related to quality of care, education, professional performance evaluation, collegiality, collaboration, ethics, research, resource utilization, and leadership.

Strategy. A plan of action to achieve a major overall goal.

Treatment adherence. The degree to which a patient complies with a healthcare provider's recommendations for care: a variety of measures including behavior can be used to measure the congruency.

REFERENCES AND RESOURCES

American Heart Association (AHA). (2007). Congenital heart disease increasingly more common in adults, children. Journal Report: 01/08/2007: Dallas: AHA.

American Heart Association (AHA). (2007). *Heart disease and stroke statistics—2007 Update*. Dallas: AHA.

American Nurses Association (ANA). (2004). *Nursing scope and standards of practice*. Washington, DC: American Nurses Publishing.

American Nurses Association (ANA). (2003). *Nursing's social policy statement*. 2nd edition. Washington, DC: Nursebooks.org.

American Nurse Association (ANA). (2002). *Nursing's agenda for the future: A call to the nation*. Washington, DC: ANA.

American Nurses Association (ANA). (2001). *Code of ethics for nursing with interpretive statements*. Washington, DC: American Nurses Publishing.

George, J. (2002). *Nursing theories: The base for professional nursing practice*. Upper Saddle River, NJ: Prentice Hall.

Institute of Medicine (IOM). (2000). *To err is human: Building a safer health system*. Washington, DC: National Academy Press.

Institute of Medicine (IOM). (2001). *Crossing the quality chasm: A new health system for the 21st century*. Washington, DC: National Academy Press.

Appendix A

Cardiovascular Nursing Associations and Societies: Missions and Websites

American Association of Cardiovascular & Pulmonary Rehabilitation
www.aacvpr.org

The mission statement of the American Association of Cardiovascular and Pulmonary Rehabilitation is to reduce morbidity, mortality, and disability from cardiovascular and pulmonary diseases through education, prevention, rehabilitation, research, and aggressive disease management.

American Association of Critical-Care Nurses (AACN)
www.aacn.org

Building on decades of clinical excellence, the American Association of Critical-Care Nurses provides and inspires leadership to establish work and care environments that are respectful, healing, and humane. The key to AACN's success is its members. Therefore, AACN is committed to providing the highest quality resources to maximize nurses' contribution to caring and improving the healthcare of acutely and critically ill patients and their families.

American Association of Heart Failure Nurses (AAHFN)
www.aahfn.org

The mission of the American Association of Heart Failure Nurses is to optimize successful outcomes for heart failure patients by uniting healthcare professionals, patients, and families in the support and advancement of heart failure practice, education, and research.

American College of Cardiology Foundation
www.acc.org

The mission of the American College of Cardiology is to advocate for quality cardiovascular care—through education, research promotion, and development and application of standards and guidelines—and to influence healthcare policy.

American College of Cardiovascular Nursing
www.accn.net

The mission of the American College of Cardiovascular Nurses is to provide evidence-based practice standards as well as primary and secondary education reflecting these standards, and to assist all levels of cardiac nurses in their preparation for Cardiovascular Nursing Board certification through online education, reference manuals, and live certification review conferences and courses.

American College of Nurse Practitioners (ACNP)
www.acnpweb.org

The mission of the American College of Nurse Practitioners is to ensure a solid policy and regulatory foundation that enables Nurse Practitioners to continue providing accessible, high-quality healthcare to the nation.

American Heart Association Council on Cardiovascular Nursing
www.americanheart.org

Building healthier lives, free of cardiovascular diseases and stroke.

Heart Failure Society of America
www.hfsa.org

The mission of the Heart Failure Society of America is to promote research related to all aspects of heart failure and to provide a forum for presentation of basic, clinical, and population-based research; educate healthcare professionals through programs, publications, and other media in the areas of basic science, clinical medicine, patient management, and social, ethical, and economic issues to enable them to diagnose and treat heart failure and concomitant medical conditions more effectively; encourage primary and secondary preventive measures to reduce the incidence of heart failure; to serve as a resource for government, private industry, and healthcare providers to facilitate the establishment of programs and policies that will better serve the patient; enhance quality and duration of life in those with heart failure; promote and facilitate the formal training of physicians, scientists, and allied healthcare providers in the field of heart failure.

Heart Rhythm Society
www.hrsonline.org

Its mission is to improve the care of patients by promoting research, education, and optimal healthcare policies and standards.

International Transplant Nurses Society

www.itns.org

The International Transplant Nurses Society is committed to the promotion of excellence in transplant clinical nursing through the provision of educational and professional growth opportunities, interdisciplinary networking and collaborative activities, and transplant nursing research.

National Association of Clinical Nurse Specialists

www.nacns.org

National Association of Clinical Nurse Specialists exists to enhance and promote the unique, high-value contribution of the clinical nurse specialist to the health and well-being of individuals, families, groups, and communities, and to promote and advance the practice of nursing.

National Gerontological Nursing Association

www.ngna.org

The National Gerontological Nursing Association's mission is to improve the quality of nursing care given to older adults.

Preventative Cardiovascular Nurses Association

www.pcna.net

The Preventive Cardiovascular Nurses Association promotes nurses as leaders in cardiovascular risk reduction and disease management.

Society of Invasive Cardiovascular Professionals

www.sicp.com

The mission of the Society of Invasive Cardiovascular Professionals is to create and maintain professional standards, promote continuing education, and act as an advocate for the nurse and technologist members of the invasive cardiovascular care team.

Society for Vascular Nursing

www.svnnet.org

The Society for Vascular Nursing's mission is to provide a professional community for vascular nursing.

Society of Pediatric Cardiovascular Nurses

www.spcnonline.com

The Society of Pediatric Cardiovascular Nurses is an international nursing organization dedicated to expanding nursing knowledge and expertise in the care of children and young adults with heart disease.

APPENDIX B.
THE SCOPE OF CARDIAC REHABILITATION PRACTICE
(1993)

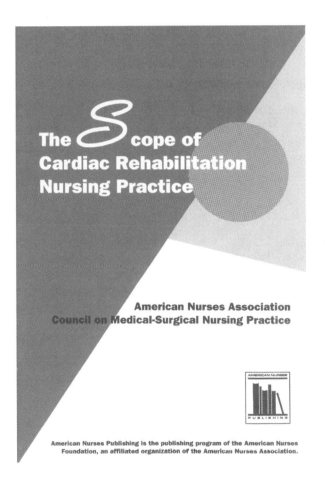

This scope document was written and developed by a task force of the American Nurses Association's Council on Medical-Surgical Nursing Practice. The Task Force on the *Scope of Cardiac Rehabilitation Nursing Practice* thanks the following reviewers who contributed comments on the document during field review—Linda Baas, M.S.N., R.N.; Kathy Berra, B.S.N., R.N., F.A.A.C.V.P.R.; Reuben Camp, R.N.; Karen Congdon, M.S., R.N.; Barbara Fletcher, M.S., R.N., F.A.A.C.V.P.R.; Erika Froelicher, Ph.D., R.N.; Sandy Harris, B.S.N., R.N.; Martha Hill, Ph.D., R.N., F.A.A.N.; Kathy Jones, B.S.N., R.N.; Nancy Phillips, M.S., R.N.; Barbara Riegel, D.N.Sc., R.N., C.S.; Eileen Stuart, M.S., R.N.; Susan Swails, B.S.N., R.N., F.A.A.C.V.P.R.; Judy Vincent, B.S.N., R.N.; and Elizabeth Winslow, Ph.D., R.N.

Task Force on the *Scope of Cardiac Rehabilitation Nursing Practice*

Cecelia Gatson Grindel Ph.D., R.N., Chair
Lehigh Valley Hospital
Allentown, Pennsylvania

Pat Comoss B.S., R.N., F.A.A.C.V.P.R.
Nursing Enrichment Consultants, Inc.
Harrisburg, Pennsylvania

Nancy Houston Miller B.S.N., R.N., F.A.A.C.V.P.R.
Stanford University
Palo Alto, California

Adele Mueller B.S., R.N.
Kennedy Memorial Hospital
Philadelphia, Pennsylvania

Judith J. Warren Ph.D., R.N.
University of Nebraska, Omaha
Omaha, Nebraska

Virginia Burggraf, M.S., R.N.
American Nurses Association
Washington, DC

Published by
American Nurses Publishing
600 Maryland Avenue, SW
Suite 100 West
Washington, DC 20024-2571

TABLE OF CONTENTS

INTRODUCTION

This book provides a statement of the scope of cardiac rehabilitation nursing practice by defining cardiac rehabilitation nursing and describing related professional role expectations. Growing demand for cardiac rehabilitation services makes such a publication timely. The increasing level of involvement by nurses in a variety of cardiac rehabilitation settings makes it appropriate.

As they have in the past, nurses will continue to be essential providers of rehabilitative care to cardiac populations. Cardiac rehabilitation nursing embraces the values and embodies the principles of *Nursing's Agenda for Health Care Reform* — i.e., individual case management, consumer self-responsibility, emphasis on healthy lifestyle, and orientation toward prevention and wellness services.[1] This scope of practice document acknowledges the past, affirms the present, and anticipates the future of cardiac rehabilitation nursing.

Service Need

The need for cardiac rehabilitation services is directly related to the prevalence of cardiovascular disease. About seven million Americans are affected by *coronary artery disease* (CAD), specifically, and, despite a dramatic decline in mortality over the last two decades, cardiovascular problems still cause more deaths each year in both men and women than all other diseases combined.[2] Over one million people survive heart attacks each year and nearly 300,000 undergo successful *coronary-artery bypass graft surgery* (CABG), and another 200,000 are treated with *percutaneous transluminal coronary angioplasty* (PTCA). These survivors are in need of services that facilitate recovery, minimize recurrence, and optimize quality of life. Programs of cardiac rehabilitation offer the structure and substance to achieve these goals.

Service Direction

Historically, cardiac rehabilitation programs have focused on secondary and tertiary prevention services, receiving patients after an acute cardiac event or a confirmed cardiac diagnosis. Though that emphasis continues today, progressive programs now serve primary prevention needs as well. They promote physical activity, good nutrition, and smoking cessation — the top three health promotion goals outlined by the U.S. Public Health Service for *Healthy People 2000: National Health Promotion and Disease Prevention Objectives*.[3]

Cardiac rehabilitation programs are as involved with shaping the health of the nation collectively as they are with optimizing cardiac patients' recoveries individually. Many are planning to expand their horizons by applying their prevention expertise across all age groups and by applying their rehabilitative strategies to other chronic disease populations.

Nursing Involvement

Cardiac rehabilitation became a separate clinical service in the late 1960s.[4] Structured rehabilitation programs offered life-restoring assistance as a follow-up to the lifesaving care provided to cardiac patients in the recently established *coronary care units* (CCUs). Nurses were involved in providing cardiac rehabilitative care then,[5-7] and have contributed substantially to the specialty's evolution ever since (see **Bibliography**).

Today, nurse researchers and clinicians continue to shape the specialty. Nurses comprise the largest group of health care professionals providing cardiac rehabilitation services in settings ranging from in-hospital, cardiac step-down units to community-based wellness programs.

Nurses are uniquely qualified to practice in cardiac rehabilitation. As licensed professionals, they are **empowered** by each of their states' nurse practice acts to provide a range of patient care services for which they are legally accountable. As registered nurses, they are **expected** by their profession to fulfill the definition of nursing expressed in *Nursing: A Social Policy Statement* — "to diagnose and treat the human responses to actual or potential health problems in the population served."[8] Through nursing education and experience, they are **enabled** to address a wide range of rehabilitation needs — from routine cardiovascular assessments to rare emergency interventions.

With this professional foundation, nurses who choose to practice in cardiac rehabilitation enhance their expertise through specialty-focused continuing education and/or advanced academic preparation. Recognizing the interdisciplinary nature of their specialty, they collaborate with physicians, exercise specialists, dietitians, physical therapists, vocational counselors, psychologists, and other health care professionals to provide cardiac rehabilitative care.

Cardiac rehabilitation nurses are involved in their own professional organization and active in interdisciplinary associations and activities pertaining to their specialty. And, they use cardiac-rehabilitation program standards produced by other professional groups (see **Contemporary Cardiac Rehabilitation Standards and Guidelines**) while adhering to their own standards of practice.[9]

PURPOSE

The purpose of cardiac rehabilitation is to assist patients with cardiovascular disease in achieving and maintaining optimal health. This assistance is provided through a partnership among nurses, patients, and/or significant others. Patients include those already medically diagnosed as having cardiovascular disease, as well as people identified as at risk for a future cardiovascular event.

The short-term goal of cardiac rehabilitation nursing is working with patients to achieve measurably positive health outcomes including minimizing physical complications, optimizing psychological recovery, aiding in the resumption of customary activities, improving functional capacity, supporting family adjustments, and promoting self-responsibility. Long-term, the goal of cardiac rehabilitative care is enabling patients to maintain a healthy lifestyle.

BELIEFS

This *Statement on the Scope of Cardiac Rehabilitation Nursing Practice* is supported by a set of beliefs and clarified by a set of definitions. Beliefs and definitions change as societal trends emerge and professions evolve.

The following list of beliefs, while not exhaustive, provides examples of important philosophical convictions which are the bases for the practice of cardiac rehabilitation nursing.

- ◆ Cardiac rehabilitation is an essential component of cardiovascular care.
- ◆ Cardiac rehabilitation is a lifelong process for the cardiovascular patient.
- ◆ Cardiac rehabilitation involves families, significant others, and other members of social support networks.
- ◆ Cardiac rehabilitation patients, as consumers of health care, have the right to expect competent, individualized care.
- ◆ Cardiac rehabilitation patients, as self-responsible adults, have the responsibility to make choices regarding their health and lifestyle.
- ◆ Nursing is an essential component of the cardiac rehabilitation process.
- ◆ Registered nurses engaged in cardiac-rehabilitation nursing practice, regardless of practice setting or educational preparation, adhere to the *Standards of Clinical Nursing Practice.*
- ◆ Cardiac rehabilitation nursing contributes significantly to enhancing the quality of life, sense of well-being, and functional status of patients with chronic cardiovascular disease.
- ◆ Cardiac rehabilitation nursing is part of an interdisciplinary health-care system.
- ◆ Cardiac rehabilitation nursing is a specialty field of practice requiring knowledge and skills beyond basic nursing preparation.
- ◆ Cardiac rehabilitation nursing addresses health promotion and prevention of disease, health restoration, and health maintenance.
- ◆ Cardiac rehabilitation nursing recognizes the biopsychosocial nature of cardiovascular disease.
- ◆ Cardiac rehabilitation nursing emphasizes understanding and adapting to chronic cardiovascular disease.
- ◆ Cardiac rehabilitation nursing empowers the patient and/or significant others helping them to make informed changes in health-related behaviors.
- ◆ Cardiac rehabilitation nursing uses available resources and innovative strategies to provide patient care.

◆ Cardiac rehabilitation nursing is based on scientific research and is supported by a substantial and growing body of knowledge and skills.

◆ Cardiac rehabilitation nursing encompasses primary, secondary, and tertiary prevention.

PRACTICE ENVIRONMENT

Cardiac-rehabilitation nursing services vary in size and by setting. Size ranges from a staff of one nurse who addresses the needs of cardiovascular clients, to large groups of nurses who function as part of an interdisciplinary team. The cardiac rehabilitation nurse is prepared through education and nursing experience to function in multiple settings. Among the more common settings are in-hospital telemetry units, ambulatory care settings (e.g., hospital-based outpatient programs, physicians' offices, free-standing clinics), community facilities (e.g., YMCA and community centers), and work-site and school-based programs.

PATIENT POPULATION

The population served by cardiac rehabilitation nurses consists of patients who have been diagnosed with cardiovascular disease or those identified as at risk for a future cardiovascular event. The population ranges widely in age, from children with congenital abnormalities to young adults experiencing single, uncomplicated cardiac events, to middle-aged patients with moderate to severe cardiovascular disease, to elderly patients with a cardiac condition complicated by other chronic disease processes. Individuals exhibiting multiple cardiovascular-risk factors also are included in this patient population.

CARDIAC REHABILITATION NURSING SERVICES

Cardiac rehabilitation services vary with the philosophy, mission, and resources of the institution. Differences in the number and type of health care providers (e.g., a single nurse or a large, interdisciplinary team) are common. Whatever the specific structure, nursing services in cardiac rehabilitation are delivered through the nursing process and are compatible with the standards of care outlined in the American Nurses Association's (ANA's) *Standards of Clinical Nursing Practice*.[8]

Services may include but are not limited to the following:

Assessment

◆ collection of health history data:

- review medical records, and,
- interview patient and family;

◆ biopsychosocial assessment:

- determine patient's awareness and perception of physical and psychological status and need for health education,
- identify cultural influences and personal values,
- identify psychological/emotional problems,
- identify usual patterns of daily living, and,
- determine patient's personal strengths and resources;

◆ physical assessment:

- perform cardiovascular examination,
- assist physician with exercise testing, and,
- compile cardiac risk profile;

◆ ongoing health assessment:

- assess changes in condition,
- evaluate new signs/symptoms,
- determine appropriateness of responses, and,
- utilize nursing judgment for appropriate action.

Diagnosis/Outcome Identification/Planning

◆ nursing care plan:

- analyze data obtained,

- derive and document nursing diagnoses,
- identify expected outcomes for specific client,
- select nursing interventions, and,
- involve patient in setting goals and priorities.

Implementation

◆ emergency care interventions:
- maintain safe, comfortable environment,
- develop written emergency plan and standing orders,
- conduct periodic emergency drills,
- maintain *Advanced Cardiac Life Support* (ACLS) certification, and,
- provide emergency care;

◆ health promotion and disease prevention:
- conduct/coordinate patient/family education,
  → develop/update cardiac lesson plans,
  → review/revise cardiac teaching aids,
  → emphasize patient's own learning priorities,
  → provide individual instruction,
  → arrange small group classes, and,
  → use appropriate written material, audiovisual aids, and other teaching strategies;
- stratify patients based on risk of future events,
  → collaborate with physician regarding prognosis,
  → identify risk status as low, moderate, or high, and,
  → assign appropriate degree of monitoring and/or supervision based on risk;
- supervise exercise program,
  → collaborate with the physician on the development of the exercise prescription,
  → conduct exercise sessions,
  → utilize exercise guidelines,
  → evaluate appropriateness of exercise response, and,
  → modify exercise plan based on principles of safe and effective exercise;
- psychosocial support,

→ provide emotional support to patient and family,

→ develop support groups for patients and families,

→ offer frequent positive reinforcement for rehabilitation progress,

→ model positive health behaviors sought from client,

→ use motivational strategies to increase program adherence;

◆ case management:

- promote continuity between inpatient and outpatient cardiac-rehabilitation programs,

- coordinate interdisciplinary rehabilitation team,

- act as patient's advocate with physician, employer, insurer, and others,

- refer to other disciplines as individually indicated for risk-factor management and/or behavior counseling, and,

- promote continuity between outpatient cardiac rehabilitation and life-long self-care;

◆ discharge planning:

Inpatient cardiac rehabilitation:

- provide discharge instructions including activity guidelines, sign/symptom recognition, and medication management, and,

- arrange referral to appropriate outpatient cardiac-rehabilitation program;

- *Outpatient cardiac rehabilitation:*

- assist patient to choose a safe, effective, realistic, follow-up exercise program to be self-managed either at home or in an appropriate community facility, or,

- arrange referral to appropriate exercise maintenance program;

◆ nursing documentation:

- maintain a chart on each patient including,

→ initial assessments upon program entry and all reassessments required by changes in the patient's condition,

→ the patient's nursing diagnoses and expected outcomes,

→ the interventions (e.g., prescriptions, protocols) planned to meet identified needs,

→ all nursing care provided,

→ the patient's response to short- and long-term outcomes of the interventions,

→ evaluation of the patient's and/or significant other's ability to manage continuing rehabilitative care after program discharge, and,

- prepare reports on patient progress and nursing performance;

Evaluation

◆ individual outcome measurement:

- collect and compare objective data from tests/measurements done at program entry and exit,
- review rehabilitative care needs noted throughout program,
- identify achievement or lack of achievement for each projected outcome,
- conduct patient/significant-other discharge interview to
  → report program results
  → request subjective feedback,
- summarize results in final written report;

◆ aggregate program effectiveness:

- distribute patient satisfaction questionnaire after program completion,
- conduct quality studies on selected nursing-care activities, and,
- track utilization of program services and explore changing trends.

EDUCATIONAL PREPARATION

The cardiac rehabilitation nurse is a licensed professional nurse prepared as a generalist. A minimum of a baccalaureate in nursing is recommended. A baccalaureate or higher degree in nursing will be required for certification as a cardiac rehabilitation nurse by the American Nurses Credentialing Center beginning in October 1994. Cardiac rehabilitation practice is not a beginning nursing position. It requires specialized knowledge and skills — including exercise adaptations and prescriptions, behavior change and motivational strategies; cardiovascular assessments and electrocardiogram (ECG) interpretation; knowledge of the pathophysiology of cardiovascular disease and current medical and surgical treatments; risk-factor reduction strategies; grounding in principles of adult education, and *advanced cardiac life support* (ACLS) capability.

Most cardiac rehabilitation nurses build their expertise on an acute cardiac-care background using a combination of self-study, continuing education seminars, specialty training courses, practice internships, on-the-job experience, and other professional activities. Those cardiac rehabilitation nurses who are credentialed in advanced nursing practice (i.e., clinical nurse specialist, nurse practitioners) expand their cardiac rehabilitation role even further to integrate professional education, research, and consultation with other patient-care services.

LEGAL ISSUES IN CARDIAC
REHABILITATION NURSING

Licensed nurses working in cardiac rehabilitation are accountable professionally and legally for their nursing practice. Since the roles and responsibilities of nurses are ever-changing and increasing in complexity, nurses must be able to make decisions regarding opportunities and limitations within their own scope of practice.

Each state licenses nurses to practice. Failure to abide by states' nurse practice acts — by neglecting a patient in need of nursing care, by practicing beyond the scope permitted by law, or by performing professional responsibilities beyond one's competence — can result in disciplinary action. Nurses in a cardiac rehabilitation setting must understand fully which services they are authorized to perform.

ETHICAL CONSIDERATIONS IN CARDIAC REHABILITATION NURSING

The importance of ethics in health care grows as society looks at health care utilization and advancing technologies. Cardiac rehabilitation nurses must apply principles of autonomy, justice, beneficence, and confidentiality when working with patients. Guided by ANA's *Code for Nurses with Interpretive Statements* [10], the cardiac rehabilitation nurse deals with a variety of ethical issues. Working with patients and other care givers, the nurse must differentiate among and clarify moral, ethical, and legal dilemmas and look for appropriate resolutions.

Several of the ethical concerns the nurse is likely to encounter involve patient participation in the cardiac rehabilitation process which:

♦ requires an informed consent process. Nurses must make sure patients fully understand and willingly consent to participate in the cardiac rehabilitation program being offered.

♦ involves the communication and documentation of extensive personal information. Patient information is to be protected without compromise in the cardiac rehabilitation setting. Confidentiality demands that such information, entrusted to a care giver, remain undisclosed.

♦ must be based on identified need. Justice demands that rehabilitation patients receive a fair distribution of the burdens and benefits of such services. Denial of access, under-utilization, over-utilization, or abuse of services, or selection of unsuitable populations for inappropriate services in cardiac rehabilitation — all challenge the ethic of justice.

♦ recognizes individual rights and responsibilities. The Patient Self-Determination Act[11] requires that all patients be provided written information concerning their involvement in treatment decisions. It is the nurse's responsibility to understand policies regarding the implementation of such rights. Nurses must know whether or not the patient has executed any advance directive and must not discriminate against an individual based on this decision. Both patients and nurses must expect that their human rights will be observed in the cardiac rehabilitation setting.

CONCLUSION

ANA recognizes the need for rehabilitative services as an essential patient-care component in the continuum of cardiac care. Because it believes that nurses are uniquely qualified to provide these services, ANA has prepared this book to specify the professional role expectations of cardiac-rehabilitation nursing practice.

ANA acknowledges the contributions other groups have made by producing standards and guidelines for cardiac rehabilitation — some in collaboration with nurses, others independently; some addressing professional competence, others focusing on program structure and operation (see **Contemporary Cardiac Rehabilitation Standards and Guidelines**). Though these publications provide various perspectives on nursing roles, only this ANA publication examines the practice of cardiac rehabilitation from the viewpoint of the nursing profession, itself.

GLOSSARY

Cardiac Rehabilitation. The process that actively assists the known cardiovascular patient in achieving and maintaining optimal health. Active assistance implies partnership among the nurses, patients, and significant others.

Cardiac Rehabilitation Nurse. A licensed professional nurse who has demonstrated expertise in cardiac-rehabilitation nursing practice, knowledge of the health problems of cardiovascular patients, and interest in helping patients achieve and maintain optimal health.

Cardiac Risk Profile. The result of the process of identifying and assessing risk factors that are easily measured, and that, either singly or in aggregate, appear to identify individuals with widely varying propensities toward the development of cardiovascular disease.

Cardiovascular Patient. An individual whose health status is affected by the diagnosis and/or treatment of coronary artery disease or other chronic cardiac or vascular problems, or a person who is at high risk for a future cardiovascular event.

Compliance. The act of conforming or adapting one's actions to another's proposal, wish, or demand.

Discharge Planning. The set of decisions and activities involved in providing continuity and coordination of care after hospitalization or completion of the outpatient phase of cardiac rehabilitation.

Exercise Guidelines. Parameters and protocols that guide cardiac-rehabilitation exercise programs.

Exercise Prescription. The specification of exercise parameters — as prescribed by the physician — involving the duration, frequency, intensity, progression, and mode of exercise.

Exercise Responses. The objective and subjective changes caused by exercise — e.g., increased heart rate and blood pressure, increased perceived exertion, increased reports of angina and/or dyspnea, and other signs/symptoms.

Exercise Testing. Exercise performed on a motor-driven treadmill, bicycle, or other ergometer with intensity gradually increasing to a medically recognized end point. Subject's heart rate, blood pressure, ECG, appearance, rate of perceived exertion, and symptoms are monitored regularly during the procedure.

Health. An optimal state of functioning in relation to one's capabilities and lifestyle, not merely the absence of disease and infirmity.

Health Education. The planning, promotion, and provision of health instruction and consultation in health-related matters.

Independent Nursing Function. Responsibility and accountability for the provision of nursing care.

Interdependent Nursing Function. Collaboration with other members of the health care team to provide patient care.

Interdisciplinary Team. A unit composed of individuals with varied and specialized training whose activities are coordinated to provide services to patients. Leadership of the team may be assigned, or it may change according to the nature of the task. The team engages in a collaborative endeavor using the combined skills and expertise of members to solve specific problems.

Intervention. An action taken by the nurse — alone or in partnership with the patient — to promote health or to treat a health problem. Nursing actions are carried out independently in the autonomous domain of nursing practice; they also may be carried out in collaboration with other health care professionals.

Liaison. An individual providing intercommunication for establishing and maintaining mutual understanding.

Modeling. The personal practice of the health behaviors that are sought from the client.

Nursing Diagnosis. A name, taxonomy label, or summarizing group of words that convey a nursing assessment conclusion regarding a client's actual or potential health problems. A nursing diagnosis involves the clinical judgment that the health or illness problem being addressed is one that the nurse has the legal authority to treat.

Patient. A program participant with whom the nurse is interacting and providing formally specified services as sanctioned by nursing practice acts.

Prevention. Health protection directed toward decreasing the probability of specific illnesses or dysfunctions in individuals, families, and communities, including active protection against unnecessary stressors.

Primary Prevention. Activities that prevent a disease from occurring.

Risk Stratification. The process of determining the likelihood of future events — based upon documented cardiovascular history — so that the most appropriate intensity of resources may be applied — i.e., the determination of the type and frequency of monitoring and supervision necessary for cardiovascular patients during rehabilitation participation.

Secondary Prevention. Activities designed to detect disease and provide early treatment (early case finding).

Tertiary Prevention. Activities engaged in by most health care providers — i.e., the treatment, care, and rehabilitation of people with acute and chronic illnesses.

Third-Party Payor. Public (e.g. Medicare, Medicaid) or private (e.g. commercial, Blue Cross) payors of health care services.

REFERENCES

1. American Nurses Association. 1991. *Nursing's Agenda for Health Care Reform*. Kansas City, Mo: American Nurses Association.

2. U.S. Department of Health and Human Services, National Center for Health Statistics. 1990. *Health, United States 1989. Prevention Profile* (Pub. No. PHS 90-1232). Washington, DC: U.S. Government Printing Office.

3. U.S. Department of Health and Human Services, Public Health Service. 1991. *Healthy People 2000 - National Health Promotion and Disease Prevention Objectives* (Pub. No. PHS 91-50213). Washington DC: U.S. Government Printing Office.

4. Berra, K.B. 1991. Cardiac and pulmonary rehabilitation: Historical perspectives and future needs. *Journal of Cardiopulmonary Rehabilitation* 11(1):8-15.

5. Lawson, M. 1972. Progressive coronary care. *Heart & Lung* (March-April):240-253.

6. Johnston, B.L., Cantwell, J.D., and Fletcher, G.F. 1976. Eight steps to inpatient cardiac rehabilitation: The team effort - Methodology and preliminary results. *Heart & Lung* (January-February):97-111.

7. Comoss, P.M., Burke, E.A.S, and Swails, S.H. 1979. *Cardiac Rehabilitation - A Comprehensive Nursing Approach*. Philadelphia: J.B. Lippincott Company.

8. American Nurses Association. 1980. *Nursing: A Social Policy Statement*. Kansas City, Mo: American Nurses Association.

9. American Nurses Association. 1991. *Standards of Clinical Nursing Practice*. Kansas City, Mo: American Nurses Association.

10. American Nurses Association. 1985. *Code for Nurses with Interpretive Statements*. Kansas City, Mo: American Nurses Association.

11. *The Patient Self-Determination Act*. PL 101-508, U.S. Congress.

CONTEMPORARY CARDIAC REHABILITATION STANDARDS AND GUIDELINES

American Association of Cardiovascular and Pulmonary Rehabilitation (AACVPR). 1991. *Guidelines For Cardiac Rehabilitation Programs.* Champaign, Ill: Human Kinetics Publishers.

Leon, A.S., Certo, C., and Comoss, P. et al. 1990. Scientific evidence of the value of cardiac rehabilitation services with emphasis on patients following myocardial infarction: Exercise conditioning component. Position paper of the AACVPR. *Journal of Cardiopulmonary Rehabilitation* (10)3:9-87.

Miller, N.H., Taylor, C.B., Davidson, D.M. et al. 1990. Position paper of the AACVPR - The efficacy of risk factor intervention and psychosocial aspects of cardiac rehabilitation. *Journal of Cardiopulmonary Rehabilitation* 10(6):198-209.

American College of Sports Medicine (ACSM). 1991. *Guidelines For Exercise Testing and Prescription.* Philadelphia: Lea and Febiger.

ACSM. 1990. Position Stand - The recommended quantity and quality of exercise for developing and maintaining cardiorespiratory and muscular fitness in healthy adults. *Medical Science Sports Exercise* 22(2):65-274.

American College of Cardiology (ACC). 1986. Position report on cardiac rehabilitation. *Journal of the American College of Cardiology* 7(2):451-453.

American College of Physicians. 1988. Position paper - Cardiac rehabilitation services. *Annals of Internal Medicine* 109:671-673.

Fletcher, G.F., Froelicher, V.F., Hartley, H. et al. 1990. Exercise standards: A statement for health professionals from the American Heart Association. *Circulation* 82(6):2136-2232.

BIBLIOGRAPHY

Selected Nursing Contributions to the Cardiac Rehabilitation Literature

Alling-Berne, L. 1987. The nurse's role: Early supervised exercise following coronary artery bypass surgery. *Focus on Critical Care* 14(6):11-16.

Berra, K. and Rudd, C.L. 1993. High-risk and special populations. In *Developing and managing cardiac rehabilitation programs,* ed. L.K. Hall. Champaign, Ill.: Human Kinetics Publishers.

Berra, K. 1991. Cardiac and pulmonary rehabilitation: Historical perspectives and future needs. *Journal of Cardiopulmonary Rehabilitation* 11(1):8-15.

Berra, K. 1992. Community resources for rehabilitation. In *Rehabilitation of the coronary patient,* 3rd ed., chap. 13, eds. N.K. Wenger and H.K. Hellerstein. New York: Churchill Livingstone, Inc.

Berra, K. 1978. Cardiac rehabilitation - Total risk factor management for persons with known coronary artery disease. *Critical Care Update* 5(10):22-27.

Berra, K.A., Fair, J.M., and Houston, N. 1977. The role of physical exercise in the prevention and treatment of coronary heart disease. *Heart & Lung* 6(2):288-292.

Berra, K.A. and Miller, N. 1981. The effects of controlled exercise on the client with coronary artery disease. *Topics in Clinical Nursing* 3(2):65-75.

Billie, D.A. 1984. Teaching the person with cardiovascular dysfunction. In *Cardiovascular nursing - Bodymind tapestry,* eds. C.E. Guzetta and B.M. Dossey. St. Louis: C.V. Mosby.

Boyd, M.D. and Citro, K. 1983. Cardiac patient education literature: Can patients read what we give them. *Journal of Cardiopulmonary Rehabilitation* 3(7):513-516.

Boyd, M.D. and Feldman, R.H.L. 1984. Health information seeking and reading comprehension abilities of cardiac rehabilitation patients. *Journal of Cardiopulmonary Rehabilitation* 4(8):343-347.

Bradley, K.M. and Williams, D.M. 1990. A comparison of the pre-operative concerns of open heart surgery patients and their significant others. *Journal of Cardiovascular Nursing* 5(1):43-53.

Bramwell, L. 1988. Social support and its relevance to cardiac rehabilitation. In *Cardiac rehabilitation nursing,* ed. C.R. Jillings. Rockville, Md: Aspen Publishers.

Budan, L.J. 1983. Cardiac patient learning in the hospital setting. *Focus on Critical Care* 10(5):16-22.

Caplin, M. 1986. Early mobilization of uncomplicated myocardial infarction patients. *Focus on Critical Care* 13(2):36-40.

Christopherson, D.J., Shively, M., and Sivarajan, E.S. 1984. Low-level exercise testing before and after coronary artery bypass surgery. *International Journal of Nursing Studies* 21(4):241-253

Comoss, P.M. 1993. Optimizing patient recovery: Inpatient cardiac rehabilitation in the 1990s. In *Critical care nursing,* chap. 69, eds. Clochesy, Breu, Cardin et al. Philadelphia: W.B. Saunders Company.

Comoss, P.M. 1992. Education of the cardiac patient and family: Principles and practice. In *Rehabilitation of the coronary patient,* 3rd ed.. eds. N.K. Wenger and H.K. Hellerstein. New York: Churchill Livingstone, Inc.

Comoss, P.M. 1988. Nursing strategies to improve compliance with life-style changes in a cardiac rehabilitation population. *Journal of Cardiovascular Nursing* 2(3):23-36.

Comoss, P.M., Burke, E.A.S., and Swails, S.H. *Cardiac rehabilitation: A comprehensive nursing approach.* Philadelphia: J.B. Lippincott Company.

Cornett, S.J. and Watson, J.E. 1984. *Cardiac rehabilitation - An interdisciplinary team approach.* New York: John Wiley and Sons.

Crosby, L.H. 1993. Issues and special populations in inpatient rehabilitation. In *Developing and managing cardiac rehabilitation programs,* ed. L.K. Hall. Champaign, Ill: Human Kinetics Publishers.

Dracup, K. et al. 1984. Family-focused cardiac rehabilitation. *Nursing Clinics of North America* 19(1):113-124.

Fletcher, B.J., Thiel, J., and Fletcher, G.F. Phase II intensive monitored cardiac rehabilitation for coronary artery disease and coronary risk factors - A six-session protocol. 1986. *American Journal of Cardiology* 57(10):751-756.

Fletcher, B.J., Lloyd A., and Fletcher, G.F.: Outpatient rehabilitative training in patients with cardiovascular disease - Emphasis on training method. *Heart & Lung* 17:2 (March) 199-205.

Fournet, K. and Schaubhut, R.M. 1986. What about spouses - SOS. *Focus on Critical Care* 13(1):14-18.

Fry, G. and Berra, K. 1981. YMCardiac therapy: Community-based cardiac rehabilitation. San Francisco: Carolyn Bean Associates.

Garding, B.S., Kerr, J.C., and Bay, K. 1988. Effectiveness of a program of information and support for myocardial infarction patients recovering at home. *Heart & Lung* 17(4):355-362.

Gerard, P.S. and Peterson, L.M. 1984. Learning needs of cardiac patients. *Cardiovascular Nursing* 20(2):7-11.

Goulart, D.T. 1989. Educating the cardiac surgery patient and family. *Journal of Cardiovascular Nursing* 3(3):1-9.

Gulanick, M. 1991. Is phase II cardiac rehabilitation necessary for early recovery of patients with cardiac disease? A randomized, controlled study. *Heart & Lung* 20(1):9-15.

Grady, K.L., Buckley, D.J., Cisar, N.S. et al. Patient perception of cardiovascular surgical patient education. *Heart & Lung* 17(4):349-355.

Hiatt, A.M., Hoenshell-Nelson, N., Zimmerman, L. 1990. Factors influencing patient entrance into a cardiac rehabilitation program. *Cardiovascular Nursing* 26(5):25-29.

Jillings, C.R. 1988. *Cardiac rehabilitation nursing.* Rockville, Md: Aspen Publishers.

Johnston, B.L.: Influence of environmental factors on exercise and activity of cardiac patients. *Cardiovascular Nursing* 18:2 (March-April 1982) 7-12.

Johnston, B.L., Watt, E.W., and Fletcher G.F. 1981. Oxygen consumption and hemodynamic and electrocardiographic responses to bathing in recent post myocardial infarction patients. *Heart & Lung* 10(4):666-671.

Karlik, B.A. and Yarcheski, A. 1987. Learning needs of cardiac patients: a partial replication study. *Heart & Lung* 16(5):544-551.

Karlik, B.A., Yarcheski, A., Braun, J., and Wu, M. 1990. Learning needs of patients with angina: An extension study. *Journal of Cardiovascular Nursing* 4(2):70-82.

Keeling, A.W. 1988. Heath promotion in coronary care and step-down units: Focus on the family - Linking research to practice. *Heart & Lung* 17(1):28-34.

Knapp, D., Hansen, M., Rogowski, B., and Pollock, M. 1985. Education of cardiac surgery patients: A comparison of the effectiveness of nurse educators and primary nurses. *Journal of Cardiopulmonary Rehabilitation* 5(9):429-434.

Lavin, M.A. 1973. Bed exercises for acute cardiac patients. *American Journal of Nursing* 73(7):1226-1227.

Lemanski, K.M. 1990. The use of self-efficacy in cardiac rehabilitation. *Progress in Cardiovascular Nursing* 5(4):114-117.

Linden, B. 1990. Unit-based phase I cardiac rehabilitation program for patients with myocardial infarction. *Focus on Critical Care* 17(1):15-19.

Livingston, M.D. 1993. Early outpatient rehabilitation. In *Developing and managing cardiac rehabilitation programs,* ed. L.K. Hall. Champaign, Ill: Human Kinetics Publishers.

Mansfield, L.W., Sivarajan, E.S., and Bruce, R.A. Exercise testing of myocardial infarction patients prior to hospital discharge: A quantitative basis for exercise prescription. *Cardiac Rehabilitation* 8:17-20.

Marshall, J.A.R. 1985. Rehabilitation of the coronary bypass patient. *Cardiovascular Nursing* 21(4):19-23.

Marshall, J.A.R. and Hawrysio, A. 1988. Inpatient recovery following myocardial infarction and coronary artery bypass graft surgery. *Journal of Cardiovascular Nursing* 2(3):1-12.

Marshall, P. 1990. Just one more - A study into the smoking attitudes and behavior of patients following first myocardial infarction. *International Journal of Nursing Studies* 27(4):375-387.

Medich, C., Stuart, E.M., Deckro, J.P., Friedman, R. 1991. Psychophysiologic control mechanisms in ischemic heart disease: The mind-heart connection. *Journal of Cardiovascular Nursing* 5(4):10-26.

Miller, N.H. Cardiac rehabilitation. In *Comprehensive cardiac care,* 7th ed., eds. Kinney, Packa, Andreoli, and Zipes. Saint Louis: Mosby Year Book, Inc.

Miller, P., Wikoff, R., Garett, M.J. et al. 1990. Regimen compliance two years after myocardial infarction. *Nursing Research* 39(6):333-336.

Miller, P. et al. 1982. Health beliefs of an adherence to medical regimen by patients with ischemic heart disease. *Heart and Lung* 11(4):332.

Murdaugh, C.L. 1988. The nurse's role in education of the cardiac patient. In *Cardiac critical care nursing,* ed. L.S. Kern. Rockville, Md: Aspen Publishers.

Murdaugh, C.L. 1982a. Using research in practice. *Focus on Critical Care* (June-July):11-14.

Murdaugh, C.L. 1982b. Barriers to patient education in the coronary care unit. *Cardiovascular Nursing* 18(6):31-36.

Murdaugh, C.L. 1980. Effects of nurses' knowledge of teaching-learning principles on knowledge of coronary care unit patients. *Heart & Lung* 9(6):1073-1078.

Newton, K.M. and Froelicher, E.S.S. 1989. Life-style adjustments. In *Cardiac nursing,* 2nd ed., eds. S.L. Underhill, S.L. Woods, E.S.S. Froelicher, and C.J. Halpenny. Philadelphia: J.B. Lippincott Company.

Newton, K.M. and Killien, M.G. 1988. Patient and spouse learning needs during recovery from coronary artery bypass. *Progress in Cardiovascular Nursing* 3(April-June):62-69.

Newton, K.M., Sivarajan, E.S., and Clarke, J.L. Patient perceptions of risk factor changes and cardiac rehabilitation outcomes after myocardial infarction. *Journal of Cardiac Rehabilitation* 5(4):159-168.

Ott, C.R. et al. 1983. A randomized study of early cardiac rehabilitation: The sickness impact profile as an assessment tool. *Heart & Lung* 12(2):162-170.

Palarski, V. and Washburn, S. 1992. Overcoming LVD in cardiac rehab. *American Journal of Nursing* (September):52-57.

Raleigh, E.H. and Odtohan, B.C. 1987. The effect of a cardiac teaching program on patient rehabilitation. *Heart & Lung* 16(3):311-317.

Riegel, B. 1988. Acute myocardial infarction - Nursing interventions to optimize supply and demand. In *Cardiac critical nursing,* ed. L.S. Kern. Rockville, Md: Aspen Publishing.

Scalzi, C.C. and Burke, L.E. 1989. Education of the patient and family: In-hospital phase. In *Cardiac nursing,* 2nd ed., eds. S.L. Underhill, S.L. Woods, E.S.S. Froelicher, and C.J. Halpenny. Philadelphia: J.B. Lippincott Company.

Sikorski, J.M. 1985. Knowledge, concerns, and questions of wives of convalescent coronary artery bypass graft surgery patients. *Journal of Cardiac Rehabilitation* 5(2):74-85.

Sivarajan, E.S. and Newton, K.M. 1984. Exercise, education, and counseling for patients with coronary artery disease. *In Symposium on cardiac rehabilitation - Clinics in sports medicine,* eds. B.A. Franklin and M. Rubenfire. Philadelphia: W.B. Saunders Company. *Clinics in Sports Medicine* 3(2):349-369.

Sivarajan, E.S., Newton, K.M., Almes, M.J., et al. 1983. Limited effects of out-patient teaching and counseling after myocardial infarction: A controlled study. *Heart & Lung* 12(1):65-73.

Sivarajan, E.S. et. al. 1982. Treadmill test responses to an early exercise program after myocardial infarction. *Circulation* 65(7):1420-1428.

Sivarajan, E.S. and Bruce, R.A. 1981. Early exercise testing after myocardial infarction. *Cardiovascular Nursing* 17(1):1-5.

Sivarajan, E.S., Bruce, R.A., Almes, M.J., Green, B., Belanger, L., Newton, K.M., and Mansfield, L.W. 1981. In-hospital exercise after myocardial infarction did not improve treadmill performance. *New England Journal of Medicine* 305(7):357-362.

Sivarajan, E.S. and Halpenny, C.J. 1979. Exercise testing. *American Journal of Nursing.* 79(12):2162-70.

Sivarajan, E.S., Valiqette Snydsman, A., Smith, B., Irving, J.B., Mansfield, L.W., and Bruce, R.A. 1977. Low-level treadmill testing of 41 patients with acute myocardial infarction prior to discharge from hospital. *Heart & Lung* 6(6):975-80.

Stanton, B.A. et al. 1984. Perceived adequacy of patient education and fears and adjustments after cardiac surgery. *Heart & Lung* 13(5):525-531.

Steele, J.M. and Ruzicki, D. 1987. An evaluation of the effectiveness of cardiac teaching during hospitalization. *Heart & Lung* 16(3):306-311.

Stuart, E.M., Caudill, M., Leserman, J., Dorrington, C., Friedman, R., and Benson, H.: Nonpharmacologic treatment of hypertension: A multiple risk factor approach. *Journal of Cardiovascular Nursing* 1(4) (August):1-14.

Thompson, D.R., Webster, R.A., and Meddis, R. 1990. Inhospital counseling for first-time myocardial infarction patients and spouses - Effects on satisfaction. *Journal of Advanced Nursing* 15(9):1064-1069.

Waitkoff, B. and Imburgia, D. 1990. Patient education and continuous improvement in a phase I cardiac rehabilitation program. *Journal of Nursing Quality Assurance* 5(1):38-48.

Wingate, S. 1990. Post MI patients' perceptions of their learning needs. *Dimensions of Critical-Care Nursing* 9(2):112-118.

Wingate, S. 1991. Acute effects of exercise on the cardiovascular system. *Journal of Cardiovascular Nursing* 5(4)(July):27-38.

Winslow, E.H. 1985. Cardiovascular consequences of bed rest. *Heart & Lung* 14(3):236-246.

Winslow, E.H. and Weber, T.M. 1980. Progressive exercise to combat the hazards of bed rest. *American Journal of Nursing* 80(3):440-445.

FIGURE 1:

Roles of the Cardiac Rehabilitation Nurse

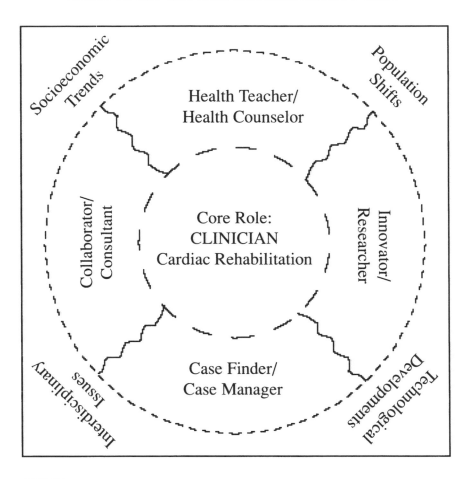

KEY:

- - - ▬ interface between core and support roles; clinical responsibilities establish nursing priorities; interface among support roles; support role emphasis shifts with demands.

- - - - interface between cardiac rehabilitation and health care environment; environmental changes have an impact on nursing roles/responsibilities.

▬▬ the health care environment; framework for cardiac-rehabilitation nursing practice.

Appendix C.
Standards of Cardiovascular Nursing Practice (1981)

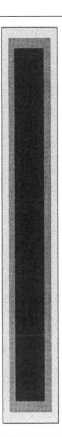

**STANDARDS
OF
CARDIOVASCULAR
NURSING PRACTICE**

**AMERICAN NURSES' ASSOCIATION
DIVISION ON MEDICAL–SURGICAL
NURSING PRACTICE
AND
AMERICAN HEART ASSOCIATION
COUNCIL ON
CARDIOVASCULAR NURSING**

These standards were approved by the Executive Committee of the American Nurses' Association Division on Medical-Surgical Nursing Practice and the Education Committee of the American Heart Association Council on Cardiovascular Nursing Practice.

Published by:

American Nurses' Association
2420 Pershing Road
Kansas City, Missouri 64108

MS-4 10M 12/81

INTRODUCTION

As the professional society for nursing in the United States, the American Nurses' Association is responsible for defining nursing, for establishing the scope of nursing practice, and for setting standards of nursing practice as a means of assuring the quality of the services nurses offer to the public.[1] A standard is an authoritative statement enunciated and promulgated by the profession by which the quality of practice can be judged.

The American Nurses' Association published *Standards of Nursing Practice* in 1973, and in 1974 published *Standards of Medical-Surgical Nursing Practice*, which had been developed by the ANA Division of Medical-Surgical Nursing Practice. Medical-surgical nursing is the nursing care of adults with known or predicted physiological alterations, with trauma, or with disability. Medical-surgical nursing practice includes the care and treatment necessary to provide comfort; to assist individuals in the promotion and maintenance of health and the prevention, detection, and treatment of illness; to promote restoration to the highest possible productive capacities; and to assist with a peaceful death.[2]

The Standards of Medical-Surgical Nursing Practice are expressed in terms of the nursing process, which includes assessment, planning, implementation, and evaluation. Because of the breadth of the scope of medical-surgical nursing practice, adaptation of the standards to several areas within medical-surgical nursing will assist nurses in the evaluation of their practice.

A joint committee of the Executive Committee of the ANA Division on Medical-Surgical Nursing Practice and the Executive Committee of the American Heart Association Council of Cardiovascular Nursing determined that standards of care for individuals who have known or predicted alterations in cardiovascular functioning would provide a means for assuring the quality of nursing care received by these individuals.

First published in 1975, the revised standards of nursing practice for care of individuals with alterations in cardiovascular functioning were jointly reviewed and expanded in 1981 by the Executive Committee of the ANA Division on Medical-Surgical Nursing Practice and the Education Committee of the AHA Council on Cardiovascular Nursing. Publication of these standards is part of the continuing work of the nursing profession to assure the quality of nursing practice.

---

[1] American Nurses' Association. *Nursing: A Social Policy Statement.* Kansas City, Mo.: the Associaton, 1980.

[2] American Nurses' Association. *A Statement on the Scope of Medical-Surgical Nursing Practice.* Kansas City, Mo.: the Association, 1980.

Appendix C: Standards of Cardiovascular Nursing Practice (1981)   **85**

STANDARDS OF CARDIOVASCULAR NURSING PRACTICE

STANDARD I

THE COLLECTION OF DATA ABOUT THE HEALTH STATUS OF THE INDIVIDUAL IS SYSTEMATIC AND CONTINUOUS. THESE DATA ARE RECORDED, RETRIEVABLE, AND COMMUNICATED TO APPROPRIATE PERSONS.

Interpretive Statement

Data are obtained by observation, interview, physical examination, review of records and reports, and consultation. Priority of data collection is determined by the immediate health care problems of the individual.

Criteria

1. Health data include, but are not limited to, the following:
   a. History regarding the following:
      1) Information about perceptions, expectations, and adherence with past prescribed and/or self-initiated dietary, medication, and activity programs
      2) Symptoms identified by the individual, including description of onset, duration, quality, location, radiation, associated symptoms, precipitating factors, relieving factors of each symptom
      3) Cardiovascular risk factor profile, including the following:
         Family history of heart disease or vascular disease
         Hypercholesterolemia/hypertriglyceridemia—serum
            lipid levels
         Smoking
         Hypertension
         Obesity
         Sedentary living
         Diabetes
         Psychosocial factors
         Alcohol intake
         Oral contraceptives
      4) Previous health state, including the following:
         Hospitalizations
         Operations
         Injuries
         Infectious diseases
      5) Personal and social factors, including the following:
         Habits
            Coffee, tea, soft drink intake

Meals
  Usual number taken daily
  Where eaten
  Description of self as "slow" or "fast" eater
Sleep
  Sleeps well/restless/poorly
  Dreams/nightmares
  Sleeps flat/upright
  Number of pillows
  Number of hours of sleep including individual's perception of adequacy
  Use of sleeping pills
Occupation
  Job description
  Physical energy expenditure
  Mental energy expenditure
  Working hours
  Shift changes
  Length of time at this work
  Job satisfaction/employer/associates
  Energy expenditure in traveling to and from work
  Chemical/physical hazards
Activities
  Hobbies
  Sports
  House/yard work
  Organizations and clubs
Living Arrangements
  Marital status
  Ages and health of spouse and children
  Number of persons in the home
  Domestic harmony/problems
Environment
  Size and arrangement of home
  Neighborhood: terrain, transportation, safety
  Pollutants
  Pets
Economic situation
  Health insurance
  Financial resources/obligations
Psychosocial readjustments
  Recent stressful life events
  Changes in role relationships
Cultural orientation, values, and beliefs
  Spiritual belief

Education
    Ability to read and understand preferred major language
    Number of years of school completed
6) Systems review
    Skin
        Diaphoresis
        Bruising
        Petechiae
    HEENT
        Headaches
        Visual problems
        Nasal stuffiness
        Allergies
        Thyroid
    Respiratory
        Cough
            Dry/productive
            Time of day/coughing at night
            Position/dependent
            Hemoptysis/secretions
        Wheezing respirations
        Dyspnea or shortness of breath
            Extertional—amount of activity that precipitates it
            Orthopnea
            Paroxysmal nocturnal dyspnea
    Cardiovascular
        Discomfort or pain in chest, arms, shoulders, back, neck, jaw
        Degree and duration of pain
        Aggravating and alleviating factors for pain
        Fatigue—change in activity tolerance
        Edema
        Claudication
        Heart consciousness
            Aware of normal heart action
            Aware of irregular beating
            Aware of pounding or palpitations
        Rheumatic fever
        Scarlet fever
        Frequent tonsillitis as a child
        "Growing pains"
        Murmur
    Gastro-intestinal
        Food preferences
        Appetite change

Food intolerance
  How manifested
  Use of antacids
Heart burn
Difficulty swallowing
Hematemesis
Stools
  Color change
  Diarrhea/constipation
Genito-urinary
  Change in urinary pattern
  Nocturia
  Hematuria
  Change in sexual desire/function
Metabolic
  Weight changes and what does individual attribute it to
Neuropsychiatric
  Dizziness
  Vertigo
  Fainting spells
    Sudden without warning
    Precipitating factors
    Fade out/grey out
  Convulsions
  Tremors
  Incoordination
  Gait changes—staggering
  Memory changes, confusion
  Changes in comprehension, understanding
  Speech changes, slurring
  Numbness, tingling
  Paralysis
Fatigue
  When noticed
  Build up during the day *vs* waking up tired
Emotional changes
  Recent mood changes
  Irritable/depressed/tense/nervous/anxious/insomnia

b. Current medical diagnosis and therapy
c. Information about previous use of and access to health services
d. Individual's psychosocial behavior and his response to illness or predicted illness/individual's expression of fears, patterns of coping/adaptation
  1) Individual's understanding of previous health problems
  2) Individual's interest in learning about health problems

e. Clincial assessment of cardiovascular functions and status in the following areas:
1) Cardiac
   Chest wall, size, configuration, and movements
   Point of maximal intensity, thrills, heaves, pulsations
   Heart sounds and murmurs
   Pericardial friction rub
   Apical/radial pulses; rate, quality, and rhythm
   Korotkoff sounds
2) Pulmonary
   Respiratory rate, quality, and pattern
   Chest expansion
   Intercostal retractions/bulging
   Position of trachea
   Diaphragm excursion
   Tactile fremitus
   Breath sounds
   Rales, rhonci, wheezes, pleural friction rub
   "E" to "A" changes, whispered pectoriloquy, brochophony
   Clubbing
3) Vascular
   Skin, color, moisture, temperature
   Petechiae
   Nailbed, mucous membrane color
   Peripheral pulses
   Homan's sign
   Blood pressure
   Pulsus alternans
   Pulsus paradoxus
   Bruits, carotid, renal artery
   Eye grounds
4) Circulatory
   Jugular venous distention
   Jugular venous pulsations
   Hepato jugular reflux
   Kussmaul's sign
   Edema
   Ascites
   Liver engorgement and enlargement
   Skin turgor
5) Effects on the neurological system
   Visual acuity
   Level of consciousness
   Restlessness
   Confusion

Syncope
Pupil response
6) Related responses
Body temperature
Xanthaloma
Arcus senilis
7) Laboratory results
Electrocardiogram
Chest x-ray
Exercise testing
CBC
Serum electrolytes
FBS
Uric Acid
Blood coagulation studies
Serum creatinine and BUN
Serum lipids
Serum enzymes
Arterial blood gases
Urine studies
2. Health data are collected by appropriate methods.
3. Health data collection is ongoing.
4. Health data includes historical summary of heatlh problems.

STANDARD II

NURSING DIAGNOSIS IS DERIVED FROM HEALTH STATUS DATA.

Interpretive Statement

The nursing diagnosis is a statement of the individual's actual or potential health problems and limitations that nurses are able to identify and treat.

Criteria

1. The nursing diagnosis identifies the individual's presenting problems and limitations.
2. Nursing diagnosis may be developed for individuals in any one of the following phases ot illness:
   a. ACUTE: occuring in response to stimuli in the immediate environment (internal and/or external) but not enduring for any length beyond the removal of those stimuli.
   b. CHRONIC: continuously present for an extended period of time.
   c. INTERMITTENT: recurring regularly at short intervals with absence of symptoms in the interim.

d. POTENTIAL: likely to occur given the combination of this person, place, and time.
3. Nursing diagnosis is derived from the following:
   a. Clinical manifestations (characteristics) of or human responses to cardiovascular problems.
   b. Hygiene, mobility, comfort, safety, sleep/rest, ventilation, circulation, nutrition, elimination, sexuality, skin integrity, prevention, and education.
   c. The recognition of the individual's unique response to each situation, e.g. diagnostic procedures, the medical therapeutic regimen, a change in lifestyle, or the use of specialized equipment.
   d. Analysis of human and community resources.
4. The nursing diagnosis provides the basis for nursing orders and should include the etiology or probable cause to ensure an appropriate treatment plan.

EXAMPLES OF NURSING DIAGNOSES	POSSIBLE ETIOLOGIES
Alteration in cardiac output	CHF, dysrhythmias, ischemic heart disease, or shock
Mobility impairment	physiological or physical limitations within the environment, e.g. being on a respirator, intra-aortic balloon pump insertion, or being on bedrest
Skin integrity impairment	mobility impairment, dehydration, invasive diagnostic tests, IV therapy, or self-care deficit
Fluid volume deficit	decreased oral intake, prolonged vomiting, diarrhea, excessive diuretic therapy, or hemorrhage
Fluid volume overload	decreased cardiac output, CHF, renal failure, excessive IV fluids, or electrolyte imbalance
Alterations in electrolyte balance	potassium deficit and excess digitalis, fluid overload, or alteration in nutrition
Sensory/perceptual alteration	excessive, insufficient, or inappropriate environmental stimuli, clinical alterations (either exogenous, e.g. drug ingestion or endogenous, e.g. electrolyte imbalance) or psychological stressors

Self-care deficit (in any or all areas of activities of daily living)	intolerance to activity, pain, perceptual cognitive impairment, neuromuscular impairment, musculo-skeletal impairment, impaired transfer ability or depression/severe anxiety
Knowledge deficit	lack of exposure, lack of recall, non-use of information, information misinterpreted, cognitive limitations, disinterest, or lack of familiarity with available resources
Non-adherence	knowledge deficit, lack of motivation, cultural/spiritual factors, fear, organic brain dysfunction, or lack of financial resources
Alteration in comfort	ischemic chest pain, myocardial infarction trauma, infection, or tension/anxiety
Sleep pattern disturbance	ischemic chest pain, fear, anxiety, environmental surroundings, or depression
Ineffective coping	situational crises, personal loss, death, illness, social changes, lack of resources, or ego fragility
Infection	invasive procedures, mobility impairment, skin integrity impairment

STANDARD III

THE PLAN OF NURSING CARE INCLUDES GOALS.

Interpretive Statement

A goal is the end state toward which nursing action is directed.

Criteria

1. Goals are derived from nursing diagnosis.
2. Goals are assigned appropriate priorities.
3. Goals are stated in terms of observable outcomes.
4. Goals are formulated by the individual, family, significant others, and health personnel.
5. Goals are congruent with the individual's present and potential physical capabilities and behavioral patterns.
6. Goals are attainable through available human and community resources.
7. Goals are achievable within an identifiable period of time.

Appendix C: Standards of Cardiovascular Nursing Practice (1981)   93

The goals of cardiovascular nursing for an individual with a known or predicted cardiovascular alteration are prevention of complications; restoration, maintenance, and promotion of optimum cardiac function; and acceptable quality of life. The following outcomes are specific to individuals with known or predicted cardiovascular alterations, but may also be applicable to any individual with any physiologic alterations. Identification of outcomes depends upon the known health status of the individual.

1. The individual is free from preventable adverse effects that may be directly related to nursing practice.
   Criteria—the individual will:
   a. Maintain cardiovascular status without further deterioration due to specific condition
   b. Be free of complications (e.g. thrombophlebitis, skin impairment, respiratory problems), due to decrease in physical activity and/or temporary maintenance of bedrest
   c. Maintain good body alignment while on bedrest to promote rest and relaxation and to decrease the workload of the heart
   d. Maintain electrolyte balance with appropriate electrolyte supplements as indicated by laboratory data to prevent cardiac complications
   e. Be free of infection at the site of insertion of invasive devices
   f. Maintain urinary output as measured every _____ hours
   g. Be free of cardiac arrhythmias due to electrical hazards
2. The individual maintains a pharmacologic regimen that is compatible with therapeutic and personal goals.
   Criteria—the individual will:
   a. Explain the rationale for the specific drug regimen prescribed
   b. State the specific action and side effects of prescribed medications
   c. Assist in determining the schedule for taking medications in the hospital or elsewhere
   d. Plan an appropriate method to assist with drug compliance in the home
3. The individual maintains an activity pattern that is compatible with therapeutic and personal goals.
   Criteria—the individual will:
   a. Explain the rationale for the specific activities prescribed
   b. State the rationale for activities to be avoided due to specific condition
   c. Develop a schedule for increasing activity and/or return to as normal a lifestyle as appropriate
   d. Evaluate tolerance to new activities based on prescribed guidelines
4. The individual maintains a dietary intake that is compatible with therapeutic and personal goals.
   Criteria—the individual will:
   a. Explain the rationale for the specific dietary regimen prescribed
   b. Maintain adequate intake of fluids as allowed

c. Maintain weight records as prescribed
5. The individual demonstrates a knowledge level that will enable modification of lifestyle.
   Criteria—the individual will:
   a. Explain the rationale for the specific therapeutic regimen prescribed
   b. Identify those factors that will promote or impede compliance
   c. Demonstrate correctly how to take radial pulse
   d. Identify symptoms due to specific disease process or therapeutic intervention that indicate the need for medical assistance
   e. Know how to obtain medical assistance
   f. Know how to obtain and use community resources
6. The individual participates in planning the modification of lifestyle and accepts the modification.
   Criteria—the individual will:
   a. State potential risk factors and relate these to own lifestyle and environment
   b. Develop a plan for modifying own risk factors within a specific period of time
7. The individual demonstrates effective coping mechanisms to adapt to his altered lifestyle.
   Criteria—the individual will:
   a. Identify coping mechanisms previously used
   b. Maintain therapeutic regimen as prescribed by the physician or nurse
   c. State the rationale for activities to be avoided due to specific condition
   d. Develop a schedule for increasing activity and/or return to as normal a life style as appropriate
   e. Evaluate tolerance to new activities based on prescribed guidelines
   f. Express feelings about specific condition and therapeutic regimen.

STANDARD IV

THE PLAN FOR NURSING CARE PRESCRIBES ACTIONS TO ACHIEVE THE GOALS.

Interpretive Statement

The determination of the results to be achieved is an essential part of planning care.

Criteria

1. The plan for nursing care is part of the multidisciplinary plan of care.
2. The plan for nursing care describes a systematic method to meet the goals.
3. The plan for nursing care is initiated following nursing diagnosis and the formulation of goals.
4. The plan for nursing care is based on current scientific knowledge of pathophysiology and phychosocial components.

5. The plan for nursing care incorporates available and appropriate material resources and environmental controls, including the following:
   a. Proper functioning of equipment
   b. Safety from electrical hazards
   c. Physical safety
   d. Noise control
   e. Humidity, temperature, and light
   f. Control of excess traffic in the clinical setting
   g. Potential and actual contaminants.
6. The plan for nursing care reflects the considerations of the "Patients Bill of Rights."*
7. The plan for nursing care specifies the following:
   a. What actions are to be performed
   b. How the actions are to be performed
   c. When the actions are to be performed
   d. Who is to perform the actions
   e. Anticipated outcomes.
8. The plan for nursing care is developed with and communicated to individual, family, significant others, and health personnel as appropriate.
9. The plan for nursing care is realistic and achievable.
10. The plan for nursing care is documented in the individual's permanent record.

STANDARD V

THE PLAN FOR NURSING CARE IS IMPLEMENTED.

Interpretive Statement

The plan is implemented to achieve the goals and is documented to enhance communication among health professionals to promote continuity of care.

Criteria

1. The nurse does one or more of the following:
   a. Provides direct care
   b. Delegates tasks and supervises the work of others
   c. Refers the individual to other professionals for specialized services
   d. Coordinates the efforts of health team members.
2. Nursing actions must:
   a. Be documented by written records
   b. Reflect the plan of care including, for example, physical ministrations, counseling, and teaching
   c. Be performed with safety, skill, and efficiency
   d. Reflect consideration of the individual's and family's dignity, beliefs, values, and desires.

*American Hospital Association, 1972

STANDARD VI

THE PLAN FOR NURSING CARE IS EVALUATED.

Interpretive Statement

The evaluation of nursing care is an appraisal of progress toward meeting the goals of care.

Criteria

1. The individual's response to nursing action is compared with the outcomes stated in the goals.
2. Information is gathered by all health care personnel involved. Examples of such information include the following:
   a. Physiologic signs, such as heart rate and rhythm, body fluid pressures, temperature, urinary output, weight, skin condition, laboratory data, and presence or absence of complications
   b. The individual's demonstrated ability to verbalize information or to perform tasks in a self-care regimen, such as drug information and self-administration, diet, activity, treatment, and a medical follow-up routine.
   c. The individual's expressed ability to cope with imposed alterations in lifestyle
   d. The individual's perceived achievement of mutually identified goals
   e. The contribution of the family and significant others to the achievement of the goals of care, including their willingness and ability to participate in and adjust to the altered lifestyle.
   f. The availability and effectiveness of human, community, and material resources utilized, including timely discharge planning and access to appropriate services.

STANDARD VII

REASSESSMENT OF THE INDIVIDUAL, RECONSIDERATION OF NURSING DIAGNOSIS, SETTING OF NEW GOALS, AND REVISION OF THE PLAN FOR NURSING CARE ARE A CONTINUOUS PROCESS.

Interpretive Statement

The steps of the nursing process are taken concurrently and recurrently.

Criteria

1. Revision of the nursing diagnosis is based on the results of the evaluation.
2. New goals formulated are consistent with the evaluation of the individual's progress and with the revised plan of care.

APPENDIX D.
STANDARDS OF CARDIOVASCULAR NURSING PRACTICE (1975)

**American
Nurses
Association**
Division on
Medical-Surgical
Nursing Practice
and
**American
Heart
Association**
Council on
Cardiovascular Nursing

*STANDARDS
of Cardiovascular
Nursing Practice*

STANDARDS
of
Cardiovascular
Nursing Practice

American Nurses Association
Division on Medical-Surgical Nursing Practice

and

American Heart Association
Council on Cardiovascular Nursing

These standards were approved by the Executive Committee of the American Nurses Association Division on Medical-Surgical Nursing Practice and the Education Committee of the American Heart Association Council on Cardiovascular Nursing Practice.

Published by
American Nurses Publishing
600 Maryland Avenue, SW
Suite 100 West
Washington, D.C. 20024-2571

First printing February 1975. Second printing and revision, December 1981. Third printing, April 1982. Fourth printing, December 1983. Fifth printing, May 1991. Sixth printing, August 1994.

CONTENTS

INTRODUCTION

As the professional society for nursing in the United States, the American Nurses Association (ANA) is responsible for defining nursing, for establishing the scope of nursing practice, and for setting standards of nursing practice as a means of assuring the quality of the services nurses offer to the public.[1] A standard is an authoritative statement enunciated and promulgated by the profession by which the quality of practice can be judged.

The American Nurses Association published *Standards of Nursing Practice* in 1973, and in 1974 published *Standards of Medical-Surgical Nursing Practice*, which had been developed by the ANA Division on Medical-Surgical Nursing Practice. Medical-surgical nursing is the nursing care of adults with known or predicted physiological alterations, with trauma, or with disability. Medical-surgical nursing practice includes the care and treatment necessary to provide comfort; to assist individuals in the promotion and maintenance of health and the prevention, detection, and treatment of illness; to promote restoration to the highest possible productive capabilities; and to assist with a peaceful death.[2]

The standards of medical-surgical nursing practice are expressed in terms of the nursing process, which includes assessment, planning, implementation, and evaluation. Because of the breadth of the scope of medical-surgical nursing practice, adaptation of the standards to several areas within medical-surgical nursing will assist nurses in the 1 evaluation of their practice.

A joint committee of the Executive Committee of the ANA Division on Medical-Surgical Nursing Practice and the Executive Committee of the American Heart Association (AHA) Council on Cardiovascular Nursing determined that standards of care for individuals who have known or predicted alterations in cardiovascular functioning would provide a means for assuring the quality of nursing care received by these individuals.

---

[1]American Nurses Association. 1980. *Nursing: A Social Policy Statement.* Kansas City, MO: the Association.

[2]American Nurses Association. 1980. *A Statement on the Scope of Medical-Surgical Nursing Practice.* Kansas City, MO: the Association.

First published in 1975, the revised standards of nursing practice for care of individuals with alterations in cardiovascular functioning were jointly reviewed and expanded in 1981 by the Executive Committee of the ANA Division on Medical-Surgical Nursing Practice and the Education Committee of the AHA Council on Cardiovascular Nursing. Publication of these standards is part of the continuing work of the nursing profession to assure the quality of nursing practice.

STANDARDS OF CARDIOVASCULAR
NURSING PRACTICE

Standard I

THE COLLECTION OF DATA ABOUT THE HEALTH STATUS OF THE INDIVIDUAL IS SYSTEMATIC AND CONTINUOUS. THESE DATA ARE RECORDED, RETRIEVABLE, AND COMMUNICATED TO APPROPRIATE PERSONS.

Interpretive Statement
Data are obtained by observation, interview, physical examination, review of records and reports, and consultation. Priority of data collection is determined by the immediate health care problems of the individual.

Criteria
1. Health data include, but are not limited to, the following:
   a. History regarding the following:
      i. Information about perceptions, expectations, and adherence with past prescribed and/or self-initiated dietary, medication, and activity programs.
      ii. Symptoms identified by the individual, including description of onset, duration, quality, location, radiation, associated symptoms, precipitating factors, relieving factors of each symptom.
      iii. Cardiovascular risk factor profile, including the following:
         * Family history of heart disease or vascular disease.
         * Hypercholesterolemia/hypertriglyceridemia — serum lipid levels.
         * Smoking.
         * Hypertension.
         * Obesity.
         * Sedentary living.
         * Diabetes.

- Psychosocial factors.
- Alcohol intake.
- Oral contraceptives.

iv. Previous health state, including the following:
- Hospitalizations.
- Operations.
- Injuries.
- Infectious diseases.

v. Personal and social factors, including the following:
- Habits
  - Coffee, tea, soft drink intake.
- Meals
  - Usual number taken daily.
  - Where eaten.
  - Description of self as "slow" or "fast" eater.
- Sleep
  - Sleeps well/restless/poorly.
  - Dreams/nightmares.
  - Sleeps flat/upright.
  - Number of pillows.
  - Number of hours of sleep, including individual's perception of adequacy.
  - Use of sleeping pills.
- Occupation
  - Job description.
  - Physical energy expenditure.
  - Mental energy expenditure.
  - Working hours.
  - Shift changes.
  - Length of time at this work.
  - Job satisfaction/employer/associates.
  - Energy expenditure in traveling to and from work.
  - Chemical/physical hazards.
- Activities
  - Hobbies.
  - Sports.
  - House/yard work.
  - Organizations and clubs.
- Living arrangements
  - Marital status.
  - Ages and health of spouse and children.
  - Number of persons in the home.
  - Domestic harmony/problems.

- Environment
  - Size and arrangement of home.
  - Neighborhood — terrain, transportation, safety.
  - Pollutants.
  - Pets.
- Economic situation
  - Health insurance.
  - Financial resources/obligations.
- Psychosocial readjustments
  - Recent stressful life events.
  - Changes in role relationships.
- Cultural orientation, values, and beliefs.
- Spiritual belief.
- Education
  - Ability to read and understand preferred major language.
  - Number of years of school completed.

vi. Systems review:
- Skin
  - Diaphoresis.
  - Bruising.
  - Petechiae.
- HEENT
  - Headaches.
  - Visual problems.
  - Nasal stuffiness.
  - Allergies.
  - Thyroid.
- Respiratory
  - Cough
    . Dry/productive.
    . Time of day/coughing at night.
    . Position/dependent.
    . Hemoptysis/secretions.
  - Wheezing respirations.
  - Dyspnea or shortness of breath
    . Exertional— amount of activity that precipitates it.
    . Orthopnea.
    . Paroxysmal nocturnal dyspnea.

- Cardiovascular
  - Discomfort or pain in chest, arms, shoulders, back, neck, jaw.
  - Degree and duration of pain.
  - Aggravating and alleviating factors for pain.
  - Fatigue — change in activity tolerance.
  - Edema.
  - Claudication.
  - Heart consciousness
    . Aware of normal heart action.
    . Aware of irregular beating.
    . Aware of pounding or palpitations.
  - Rheumatic fever.
  - Scarlet fever.
  - Frequent tonsillitis as a child.
  - "Growing pains."
  - Murmur.
- Gastrointestinal
  - Food preferences.
  - Appetite change.
- Food intolerance
  - How manifested.
  - Use of antacids.
- Heartburn.
- Difficulty swallowing.
- Hematemesis.
- Stools
  - Color change.
  - Diarrhea/constipation.
- Genitourinary
  - Change in urinary pattern.
  - Nocturia.
  - Hematuria.
  - Change in sexual desire/function.
- Metabolic
  - Weight changes and what does individual attribute it to.
- Neuropsychiatric
  - Dizziness.
  - Vertigo.
  - Fainting spells
    . Sudden, without warning.

. Precipitating factors.
. Fade out/grey out.
- Convulsions.
- Tremors.
- Incoordination.
- Gait changes — staggering.
- Memory changes, confusion.
- Changes in comprehension, understanding.
- Speech changes, slurring.
- Numbness, tingling.
- Paralysis.
- Fatigue
  - When noticed.
  - Build up during the day vs. waking up tired.
- Emotional changes
  - Recent mood changes.
  - Irritable/depressed/tense/nervous/anxious/insomnia.
b. Current medical diagnosis and therapy.
c. Information about previous use of and access to health services.
d. Individual's psychosocial behavior and his/her response to illness or predicted illness; individual's expression of fears, patterns of coping/adaption:
  i. Individual's understanding of previous health problems.
  ii. Individual's interest in learning about health problems.
e. Clinical assessment of cardiovascular functions and status in the following areas:
  i. Cardiac
    - Chest wall, size, configuration, and movements.
    - Point of maximal intensity, thrills, heaves, pulsations.
    - Heart sounds and murmurs.
    - Pericardial friction rub.
    - Apical/radial pulses; rate, quality, and rhythm.
    - Korotkoff sounds.
  ii. Pulmonary
    - Respiratory rate, quality, and pattern.
    - Chest expansion.
    - Intercostal retractions/bulging.
    - Position of trachea.
    - Diaphragm excursion.

- Tactile fremitus.
- Breath sounds.
- Rales, rhonchi, wheezes, pleural friction rub.
- "E" to "A" changes, whispered pectoriloquy, bronchophony.
- Clubbing.

iii. Vascular
- Skin, color, moisture, temperature.
- Petechiae.
- Nailbed, mucous membrane color.
- Peripheral pulses.
- Homan's sign.
- Blood pressure.
- Pulsus alternans.
- Pulsus paradoxus.
- Bruits, carotid, renal artery.
- Eye grounds.

iv. Circulatory
- Jugular venous distention.
- Jugular venous pulsations.
- Hepato jugular reflux.
- Kussmaul's sign.
- Edema.
- Ascites.
- Liver engorgement and enlargement.
- Skin turgor.

v. Effects on the neurological system
- Visual acuity.
- Level of consciousness.
- Restlessness.
- Confusion.
- Syncope.
- Pupil response.

vi. Related responses
- Body temperature.
- Xanthaloma.
- Arcus senilis.

vii. Laboratory results
- Electrocardiogram.
- Chest x-ray.
- Exercise testing.
- CBC.

- Serum electrolytes.
- FBS.
- Uric acid.
- Blood coagulation studies.
- Serum creatinine and BUN.
- Serum lipids.
- Serum enzymes.
- Arterial blood gases.
- Urine studies.

2. Health data are collected by appropriate methods.
3. Health data collection is ongoing.
4. Health data includes historical summary of health problems.

Standard II

NURSING DIAGNOSIS IS DERIVED FROM HEALTH STATUS DATA.

Interpretive Statement

The nursing diagnosis is a statement of the individual's actual or potential health problems and limitations that nurses are able to identify and treat.

Criteria
1. The nursing diagnosis identifies the individuals presenting problems and limitations.
2. Nursing diagnosis may be developed for individuals in any one of the following phases of illness:
   a. <u>Acute</u> — Occurring in response to stimuli in the immediate environment (internal and/or external) but not enduring for any length beyond the removal of those stimuli.
   b. <u>Chronic</u> — Continuously present for an extended period of time.
   c. <u>Intermittent</u> — Recurring regularly at short intervals with absence of symptoms in the interim.
   d. <u>Potential</u> — Likely to occur given the combination of this person, place, and time.
3. Nursing diagnosis is derived from the following:
   a. Clinical manifestations (characteristics) of or human responses to cardiovascular problems.
   b. Hygiene, mobility, comfort, safety, sleep/rest, ventilation, circulation, nutrition, elimination, sexuality, skin integrity, prevention, and education.

c. Recognition of the individual's unique response to each situation — e.g., diagnostic procedures, the medical therapeutic regimen, a change in lifestyle, or the use of specialized equipment.
d. Analysis of human and community resources.
4. The nursing diagnosis provides the basis for nursing orders and should include the etiology or probable cause to ensure an appropriate treatment plan.

Examples of Nursing Diagnoses	Possible Etiologies
• Alteration in cardiac output	CHF, dysrhythmias, ischemic heart disease, or shock
• Mobility impairment	Physiological or physical limitations within the environment — e.g., being on a respirator, intra-aortic balloon pump insertion, or being on bedrest
• Skin integrity impairment	Mobility impairment, dehydration, invasive diagnostic tests, IV therapy, or self-care deficit
• Fluid volume deficit	Decreased oral intake, prolonged vomiting, diarrhea, excessive diuretic therapy, or hemorrhage
• Fluid volume overload	Decreased cardiac output, CHF, renal failure, excessive IV fluids, or electrolyte imbalance
• Alterations in electrolyte balance	Potassium deficit and excess digitalis, fluid overload, or alteration in nutrition
• Sensory/perceptual alteration	Excessive, insufficient, or inappropriate environmental stimuli, clinical alterations (either exogenous — e.g., drug ingestion — or endogenous — e.g., electrolyte imbalance), or psychological stressors

• Self-care deficit (in any or all areas of activies of daily living)	Intolerance to activity, pain, perceptual cognitive impairment, neuromuscular impairment, musculoskeletal impairment, impaired transfer ability or depression/severe anxiety
• Knowledge deficit	Lack of exposure, lack of recall, nonuse of information, information misinterpreted, cognitive limitations, disinterest, or lack of familiarity with available resources
• Non-adherence	Knowledge deficit, lack of motivation, cultural/spiritual factors, fear, organic brain dysfunction, or lack of financial resources
• Alteration in comfort	Ischemic chest pain, myocardial infarction trauma, infection, or tension/anxiety
• Sleep pattern disturbance	Ischemic chest pain, fear, anxiety, environmental surroundings, or depression
• Ineffective coping	Situational crises, personal loss, death, illness, social changes, lack of resources, or ego fragility
• Infection	Invasive procedures, mobility impairment, skin integrity impairment

Standard III

THE PLAN OF NURSING CARE INCLUDES GOALS.

Interpretive Statement
A goal is the end state toward which nursing action is directed.

Criteria
1. Goals are derived from nursing diagnosis.
2. Goals are assigned appropriate priorities.
3. Goals are stated in terms of observable outcomes.
4. Goals are formulated by the individual, family, significant others, and health personnel.
5. Goals are congruent with the individual's present and potential physical capabilities and behavioral patterns.
6. Goals are attainable through available human and community resources.
7. Goals are achievable within an identifiable period of time.

Examples of Goals of Nursing Care

The goals of cardiovascular nursing for an individual with a known or predicted cardiovascular alteration are prevention of complications; restoration, maintenance, and promotion of optimum cardiac function; and acceptable quality of life. The following outcomes are specific to individuals with known or predicted cardiovascular alterations, but also may be applicable to any individual with any physiologic alterations. Identification of outcomes depends upon the known health status of the individual.
1. The individual is free from preventable adverse effects that may be directly related to nursing practice.

Criteria
The individual will:
a. Maintain cardiovascular status without further deterioration due to specific condition.
b. Be free of complications (e.g., thrombophlebitis, skin impairment, respiratory problems) due to decrease in physical activity and/or temporary maintenance of bedrest.
c. Maintain good body alignment while on bedrest to promote rest and relaxation and to decrease the workload of the heart.
d. Maintain electrolyte balance with appropriate electrolyte supplements as indicated by laboratory data to prevent cardiac complications.
e. Be free of infection at the site of insertion of invasive devices.
f. Maintain urinary output as measured every __ hours.
g. Be free of cardiac arrhythmias due to electrical hazards.

2. The individual maintains a pharmacologic regimen that is compatible with therapeutic and personal goals.

Criteria
   The individual will:
   a. Explain the rationale for the specific drug regimen prescribed.
   b. State the specific action and side effects of prescribed medications.
   c. Assist in determining the schedule for taking medications in the hospital or elsewhere.
   d. Plan an appropriate method to assist with drug compliance in the home.
3. The individual maintains an activity pattern that is compatible with therapeutic and personal goals.

Criteria
   The individual will:
   a. Explain the rationale for the specific activities prescribed.
   b. State the rationale for activities to be avoided due to specific condition.
   c. Develop a schedule for increasing activity and/or returning to as normal a lifestyle as appropriate.
   d. Evaluate tolerance to new activities based on prescribed guidelines.
4. The individual maintains a dietary intake that is compatible with therapeutic and personal goals.

Criteria
   The individual will:
   a. Explain the rationale for the specific dietary regimen prescribed.
   b. Maintain adequate intake of fluids as allowed.
   c. Maintain weight records as prescribed.
5. The individual demonstrates a knowledge level that will enable modification of lifestyle.

Criteria
   The individual will:
   a. Explain the rationale for the specific therapeutic regimen prescribed.
   b. Identify those factors that will promote or impede compliance.

c. Demonstrate correctly how to take radial pulse.
   d. Identify symptoms due to specific disease process or
      therapeutic intervention that indicate the need for medi-
      cal assistance.
   e. Know how to obtain medical assistance.
   f. Know how to obtain and use community resources.
6. The individual participates in planning the modification of
   lifestyle and accepts the modification.

Criteria
   The individual will:
   a. State potential risk factors and relate these to own
      lifestyle and environment.
   b. Develop a plan for modifying own risk factors within a
      specific period of time.
7. The individual demonstrates effective coping mechanisms to
   adapt to his/her altered lifestyle.

Criteria
   The individual will:
   a. Identify coping mechanisms previously used.
   b. Maintain therapeutic regimen as prescribed by the physi-
      cian or nurse.
   c. State the rationale for activities to be avoided due to
      specific condition.
   d. Develop a schedule for increasing activity and/or return-
      ing to as normal a lifestyle as appropriate.
   e. Evaluate tolerance to new activities based on prescribed
      guidelines.
   f. Express feelings about specific condition and therapeutic
      regimen.

Standard IV

THE PLAN FOR NURSING CARE PRESCRIBES ACTIONS TO ACHIEVE THE
GOALS.

Interpretive Statement
   The determination of the results to be achieved is an essential
part of planning care.

Criteria
1. The plan for nursing care is part of the multidisciplinary plan of care.
2. The plan for nursing care describes a systematic method to meet the goals.
3. The plan for nursing care is initiated following nursing diagnosis and the formulation of goals.
4. The plan for nursing care is based on current scientific knowledge of pathophysiology and psychosocial components.
5. The plan for nursing care incorporates available and appropriate material resources and environmental controls, including the following:
   a. Proper functioning of equipment.
   b. Safety from electrical hazards.
   c. Physical safety.
   d. Noise control.
   e. Humidity, temperature, and light.
   f. Control of excess traffic in the clinical setting.
   g. Potential and actual contaminants.
6. The plan for nursing care reflects the considerations of the "Patient's Bill of Rights."*
7. The plan for nursing care specifies the following:
   a. What actions are to be performed.
   b. How the actions are to be performed.
   c. When the actions are to be performed.
   d. Who is to perform the actions.
   e. Anticipated outcomes.
8. The plan for nursing care is developed with and communicated to the individual, family, significant others, and health personnel as appropriate.
9. The plan for nursing care is realistic and achievable.
10. The plan for nursing care is documented in the individual's permanent record.

---

* American Hospital Association. 1972. "Statement On a Patient's Bill of Rights." Chicago, IL: the Association.

Standard V

THE PLAN FOR NURSING CARE IS IMPLEMENTED.

Interpretive Statement
The plan is implemented to achieve the goals and is documented to enhance communication among health professionals to promote continuity of care.

Criteria
1. The nurse does one or more of the following:
   a. Provides direct care.
   b. Delegates tasks and supervises the work of others.
   c. Refers the individual to other professionals for specialized services.
   d. Coordinates the efforts of health team members.
2. Nursing actions must:
   a. Be documented by written records.
   b. Reflect the plan of care—including, for example, physical ministrations, counseling, and teaching.
   c. Be performed with safety, skill, and efficiency.
   d. Reflect consideration of the individual's and family's dignity, beliefs, values, and desires.

Standard VI

THE PLAN FOR NURSING CARE IS EVALUATED.

Interpretive Statement
The evaluation of nursing care is an appraisal of progress toward meeting the goals of care.

Criteria
1. The individual's response to nursing action is compared with the outcomes stated in the goals.
2. Information is gathered by all health care personnel involved. Examples of such information include the following:
   a. Physiologic signs, such as heart rate and rhythm, body fluid pressures, temperature, urinary output, weight, skin condition, laboratory data, and presence or absence of complications.

    b. The individual's demonstrated ability to verbalize information or to perform tasks in a self-care regimen, such as drug information and self-administration, diet, activity, treatment, and a medical follow-up routine.

    c. The individual's expressed ability to cope with imposed alterations in lifestyle.

    d. The individual's perceived achievement of mutually identified goals.

    e. The contribution of the family and significant others to the achievement of the goals of care, including their willingness and ability to participate in and adjust to the altered lifestyle.

    f. The availability and effectiveness of human, community, and material resources utilized, including timely discharge planning and access to appropriate services.

Standard VII

REASSESSMENT OF THE INDIVIDUAL, RECONSIDERATION OF NURSING DIAGNOSIS, SETTING OF NEW GOALS, AND REVISION OF THE PLAN FOR NURSING CARE ARE A CONTINUOUS PROCESS.

Interpretive Statement

The steps of the nursing process are taken concurrently and recurrently.

Criteria

1. Revision of the nursing diagnosis is based on the results of the evaluation.

2. New goals formulated are consistent with the evaluation of the individual's progress and with the revised plan of care.

INDEX

An index entry preceded by a bracketed calendar year indicates an entry from a previous edition or predecessor publication that is included in this edition as an appendix. Thus: [1993] is *Scope of Cardiac Rehabilitation Nursing* (Appendix B); [1981] is *Standards of Cardiovascular Nursing Practice* (Appendix C); and [1975] is *Standards of Cardiovascular Nursing Practice* (Appendix D).

American Nurses Association
(*continued*)
  *Standards of Medical-Surgical Nursing
    Practice*, 103
  Standards of Nursing Practice, 103
    [1993], 53, 55
American Nurses Credentialing Center
    (ANCC), 9, 65
Analysis. *See* Critical thinking, analysis,
    and synthesis
Arrhythmia, xi, 6
Assessment, 3, 58
  cardiovascular, 2, 5, 65
  criteria, 8, 15
  data collection for, 15
    [1981], 86–91
    [1975], 105–111
  data used in diagnosis, 16
  defined, 41, 42
  diagnosis and, 16, 19, 25
  evaluation and, 16
  as nursing process step, 15–16, 19
  as nursing service [1993], 61–62
  reassessment standard of care
    [1981], 97
    [1975], 119
  skills, 6
  standard of practice, 6–9
  See also Data collection
Atrial fibrillation, 3

C
Cardiac rhythm managing devices, 6
Cardiac rehabilitation nurse [1993], 4
  assessment, 59
  beliefs, 55–56
  case management, 60, 63
  defined, 55, 65, 69
  diagnosis, 59, 61–62
  disease prevention, 55–56
  documentation, 63
  education, 55, 57
  ethics, 67
  evaluation, 59, 64
  glossary of terms, 69–71
  health promotion, 55
  history, 53

implementation, 63–64
intervention, 59, 63
knowledge base, 59
legal issues, 66
nursing services, 61–64
outcomes identification, 59, 61–62
patient population, 58
planning, 59, 61–62, 63
  [1981], 93–95
practice environment, 57, 59
prescriptive authority and treatment,
  65
purpose, 54
research, 56, 59
roles of, 59–60, 81
services, 52, 61–64
strategies, 52
terminology, 69–71
Cardiovascular assessment, 65
Cardiovascular disease, xi, 1–3, 12
  arrythmia, xi, 6
  chronic, 2
  definition, xi
  detecting, 1
  epidemiology, 2
  pathophysiology, 2, 65
  preventing, xii, 1, 2, 8, 12, 13
  treating, 1, 7–8
  [1993], 52–53
Cardiovascular health, 1
  education, 1, 6, 8, 12, 13, 16, 22, 35
  interventions, 1, 6
  plan, 18–19
  risk factors, 16
    [1981], 86
    [1975], 105
Cardiovascular nursing
  assessment, 2, 3, 5, 15–16
  body of knowledge, 6–7, 13, 29
  certification, 9–10, 27, 28, 29
    [1993], 62, 65
  characteristics, 3–4
  collaboration, 32
  collegiality, 31
  consultation, 23
  data (health data) collection, 15, 34
  defined, 1–2, 39

Coordination of care (*continued*)
[1993], 52, 63
See also Interdisciplinary health care
Coronary artery disease (CAD), 3
[1993], 52
Coronary-artery bypass surgery (CABG)
[1993], 52
Coronary care units (CCUs), xi
[1993], 53
Cost control, xi, 8, 12, 28, 40
coordination of care and, 24, 35
outcomes identification and, 17
planning and, 35
quality of practice and, 28
resource utilization and, 35
Cost-effectiveness. *See* Cost control
Credentialing. *See* Certification and
credentialing
Criteria. *See* Measurement criteria
Critical thinking, analysis, and
synthesis, 3, 7
planning and, 19
synthesis of data and information, 21

D
Data (defined), 39
Data collection, 15, 27, 34
[1981], 86–90
[1975], 105–111
See also Assessment
Data and information usage and
synthesis, 16, 21
Decision-making, 6, 11, 12, 18, 34, 40,
41, 42
collaboration and, 32
consultation and, 23
leadership and, 36–37
professional practice evaluation and,
30
Diagnosis, 6–8, 41, 42
defined, 39
as nursing process step, 20, 25
as nursing service [1993], 61–62
standard of practice, 16
[1981], 92–93
[1975], 111–113
tools, 6

Disease management , 1, 2, 6
defined, 39–40
Documentation, 3, 25
collaboration and, 32
coordination of care and, 21, 27
diagnosis and, 18
evaluation and, 25
[1993], 63
planning and, 32
[1981], 96
quality of practice and, 27
Dysrhythmia recognition, 6

E
Economic issues. *See* Cost control
Education of cardiovascular nurses, 1,
4–8, 29
advanced requirements, 7–8
credentialing and, 4–5
general requirements, 4–7
[1993], 55, 57
See also Mentoring; Professional
development
Education of patients and families, 1, 6,
8, 12, 13, 16, 35
See also Family; Health teaching and
health promotion; Patient
Elderly population, 4, 16
Electrophysiology, 6
Electrocardiogram (ECG), 65
Environment (of practice/work; defined),
40
See also Practice environment
Ethics, 6, 11, 17, 27
code of (defined), 39
code for nurses, 33, 43, 67
standard of professional performance,
33, 42
[1993], 67
Evaluation, 9, 11
defined, 40, 42
health teaching and health
promotion, 22
as nursing process step, 30
as nursing service [1993], 64
resource utilization and, 35
standard of practice, 17, 22, 25, 35

Interdisciplinary health care (*continued*)
case management, 6
communication, 11
ethics and, 33
leadership and, 36–37
quality of practice and, 28
See also Collaboration; Healthcare
providers; Multidisciplinary health
care
International Transplant Nurses Society,
47
Internet, 45–47

K
Knowledge (defined), 41
Knowledge base
cardiovascular nursing, 6–7, 13, 29
cardiovascular rehabilitation nursing
[1993], 59

L
Laws, statutes, and regulations, 24
evaluation and, 25
planning and, 18
professional practice evaluation and,
30
[1993], 66
Leadership, 8, 21, 45
standard of professional performance,
36, 42
See also Mentoring
Licensing. *See* Certification and
credentialing
Long-term care, 12, 16

M
Measurement criteria
advanced practice nurse, 15–16
assessment, 8, 15
collaboration, 1, 32
collegiality, 31
consultation, 23
coordination of care, 21, 2
defined (as criteria) , 39
diagnosis, 16,
education, 29
ethics, 33

evaluation, 25
health data collection
[1975], 105–111
[1981], 86–91
health teaching and health promotion,
22
implementation, 20
leadership, 36–37
outcomes identification, 17
planning, 18–19
prescriptive authority and treatment,
24
professional practice evaluation, 30
quality of practice, 27–28
research, 34
resource utilization, 20, 35
See also entries for each Standards of
practice; Standards of professional
performance
Mentoring, 34
collegiality and, 31
leadership and, 36
See also Education of cardiovascular
nurses; Professional development
Multidisciplinary (defined), 41
Multidisciplinary health care, 6, 7, 17, 18,
21, 31, 32, 35
See also Collaboration; Healthcare
providers; Interdisciplinary health
care

N
National Association of Clinical Nurse
Specialists, 47
National Gerontological Nursing
Association, 47
Nurse (defined), 41
Nurse Practitioner (NP), 7–8
[1993], 65
Nursing (defined), 41
Nursing care standards.
See also Standards of care
Nursing process, 6
assessment as step, 15–16, 19, 61
diagnosis as step, 20, 25, 64
evaluation as step, 30, 64
implementation as step, 17

nursing services and [1993], 61
outcomes identification as step, 18
quality of practice and, 27
See also Assessment; Diagnosis;
   Evaluation; Implementation;
   Planning; Outcomes identification
Nursing services in cardiac rehabilitation
   [1993], 61–64
Nursing standards. *See* Standards of
   practice; Standards of professional
   performance

O
Outcomes, 11–12, 20, 23, 36–37, 41, 45
  collaboration and, 32
  defined, 41
  diagnosis and, 16, 39
    [1993], 61–62
  ethics and, 33
  evaluation and, 25, 40
  planning and, 18, 41
  quality of practice and, 17, 42
  See also Outcomes identification
Outcomes identification
  defined, 17
  as nursing process step, 18
  as nursing service with diagnosis [1993],
    61–62
  as planning goal standard, 93, 113–
    116
  standard of practice, 17
    [1981], 93
    [1975], 113–116
  See also Outcomes

P
Pacemakers, 10
Palliative procedure, xi
Parents. See Family
Patient, xi, 1–2, 5–12, 34–35
  assessment and, 15
    [1981], 87–91
  Bill of Rights, 96, 117
  collaboration and, 32
  collegiality and, 32
  consultation, 23
  coordination of care and, 21

defined, 41
  [1993], 70
diagnosis and, 16
ethics and, 33
  [1993], 67
evaluation, 29–30
health teaching and health promotion,
  22
monitoring systems, 6
outcomes identification and, 1, 8, 17
Patient Self-Determination Act, 67
planning, 18–19
population, 3–4
  [1993], 58
satisfaction, 1
Patient Self-Determination Act, 67
  See also Education of patients and
    families; Family
Peer review, 30
  defined, 41
Pharmacologic therapies, 7–8, 24
  adverse effects, 24
  prescriptive authority standard, 24
Pharmacogenomics, 10
Planning, 1, 9, 11–12, 39, 41
  collaboration and, 32
  consultation and, 23
  defined (as Plan), 41
  diagnosis and, 16
    [1993], 61–62
  evaluation and, 25
    [1975], 118–119
  implementation and, 20, 40
    [1981], 97
    [1993], 63
  leadership and, 36
  as nursing process step, 18
  as nursing service [1993], 61–62
  outcomes identification and, 17
  resource utilization and, 35
  standard of practice, 18–19, 42
    [1975], 113–119
    [1981], 95–97
Policy. See Healthcare policy
Practice environment, xi, 1, 4, 5, 9–11, 15,
  40, 41, 45
  assessment and, 28

Practice environment (*continued*)
  education and, 31
  leadership and, 36
  in measurement criteria, 17, 18, 21, 28
    [1993], 57, 59
Practice-based research, 1, 40
Practice roles. *See* Roles in cardio-
    vascular nursing practice
Practice settings. *See* Practice
    environment
Preceptors. *See* Mentoring
Prescriptive authority and treatment, 8
  standard of practice, 24
    [1993], 65
Preventive Cardiovascular Nurses
    Association, 47
Privacy. *See* Confidentiality
Professional development, 8–9
  cardiovascular nursing
  education and, 8–9
  See also Education; Leadership;
    Mentoring
Professional organizations, 36
  See also American Heart Association;
    American Nurses Association; *other*
    American ... *and* Society ... *entries*
Professional performance. *See* Standards
    of professional performance
Professional practice evaluation
  standard of professional performance,
    30

Q
Quality of care (defined), 41
Quality of life, 12
  defined, 42
    [1993], 56
Quality of practice, 41
  improvements, 27, 28
  standard of professional performance,
    27–28, 42

R
Recipient of care (defined), 41
  See also Patient
Referrals. *See* Collaboration; Coordination
  of care

Registered Nurse (RN), 1, 4, 11
Regulatory issues. *See* Laws, statutes,
    and regulations
Research, 1–4, 7–8, 11, 45–47
  assessment and, 28
  collaboration and, 32
  consultation and, 23
  education and, 29
  ethics and, 33
  generating, 28
  planning and, 18–19
  practice-based, 1, 40
  quality of practice, 28
  standard of professional performance,
    34, 42
    [1993], 56, 59
  See also Evidence-based practice
Resource utilization, 6, 10, 12, 18, 21, 39
  health teaching and health promotion,
    22
  implementation and, 20
  standard of professional performance,
    35, 42
Risk assessment, 8
Risk factors in cardiovascular health, 10, 16
    [1981], 86
    [1975], 105
Roles in cardiac rehabilitation nursing,
    59–60, 81
Roles in cardiovascular nursing practice,
    3–4
  See also Advanced practice
    cardiovascular nursing; Advanced
    Practice Registered Nurse; Clinical
    Nurse Specialist; Registered Nurse

S
Scientific findings. *See* Evidence-based
    practice; Research
Scope of practice of cardiac rehabilitation
    nursing [1993], 49–71
Scope of practice of cardiovascular
    nursing, 1–13
    [1975], 103
Self care and self management, 1–3, 9,
    12, 22, 33
  defined, 42

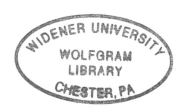